I Can and I Will

Cultivate Your Courage for the Natural Birth of Your Dreams

WENDY HANENBURG

To my sweet children, Griffin and Ainsley, who still inspire me to find my courage, and to my wonderful husband, David, for his encouraging support during the natural births of our children as well as in life.

Thank you for being you!

People must remind each other that it can be done, and it must be done. We must keep up each other's courage. In that way, we are enormously strong.

-Vincent van Gogh

CONTENTS

INTRODUCTION

Nobody can give you courage. You already have your own courage; it's inside you. But you may need someone to remind you and inspire you. Especially at an important time such as this.

Congratulations! You are probably expecting a baby, or are planning to have a baby in the near future. I bet there are so many feelings running through you right now: Excitement. Wonder. Awe.

Apprehension.

Curiosity.

There's a spark inside you.

You want to know more about natural birth: specifically, "Can I do it?" and especially, "How do I do it?"

It is intriguing in this day and age, isn't it? The thought of someone purposely choosing to experience labor pain when they don't have to.

We hear stories about natural birth. Few and far between, perhaps, but they are out there. Softly spoken words find their way to our ears: ...amazing...empowering...healthier...joy...ecstatic...important.

Can those words really be spoken about birth? That supposedly dreadful experience we have to suffer through as a woman if we want to have a baby? What is there of this JOY? Joy because your baby is here, yes. But joy because of the process of getting the baby here? Interesting...

So here you are, wanting a natural birth. Ready to jump in. (Or tip-toe in. Your call.) Ready for some JOY.

Does this sound familiar? You want to have a natural childbirth but don't know who you can talk to for support and encouragement, or where you can get information to help you get through it.

I can help you go from, "I want to have a natural childbirth" to "I birthed my baby naturally – and it was awesome!"

I will show you that any woman who wants to experience natural childbirth can indeed do so.

It IS possible. You CAN do this!

Who am I?

How am I qualified to help someone achieve the natural birth of her dreams?

My name is Wendy Hanenburg and I birthed both my babies naturally. My son was born in a freestanding birth center and my daughter was born at home, both with a midwife attending. I am not a midwife, doctor, doula, nurse, childbirth educator, or in any area of the health care industry. (In fact, my college degree was in Electrical Engineering.)

I am a regular woman just like you. I have a wide variety of interests, ranging from musical (I learned to play the drums two years ago; Foo Fighters is my favorite band) to crafty (I like sewing projects and creating party invitations and decorations) to natural (organic food, natural health, breastfeeding, natural birth).

If you had told me 15 years ago that I would birth my babies naturally—and with a midwife attending, no less—I would have laughed! (Politely, of course.) I used to cite my "low pain tolerance" for the reason I assumed I would choose an epidural when it was time to have a baby. (Really. Any stubbed toe or bonked elbow will have me howling in pain and practically curled in a ball.)

How did I get from there to here?

Being a reader and planner, I started learning about birth years before I was even pregnant. The **knowledge** I gained about birth led to a **belief** in my ability as well as to a strong **determination** to have a natural birth, which in turn led to choosing a **supportive** caregiver and **planning** for a natural birth.

These five keys to natural birth all worked together in a symbiotic way and interesting things happened to this self-described "low pain tolerance", want-to-be-in-control, Type A planner:

     ** I learned to trust birth.
     ** I learned to trust my body.
     ** I learned to trust my baby.
     ** **I found my courage**.

I found *my* courage. I had it all along. I just needed to tap into it.

The paradigm of my ideal birth shifted from one where I wanted to avoid all sensation, to one where I wanted to feel everything about this **unique opportunity of bringing a baby into the world**.

And once my baby was born naturally I was ecstatic! I felt strong. I felt empowered. I felt joy. It was almost a surprise, even after all that planning.

Really? Giving birth can feel that great?!

It was such an amazing experience and **I want that same experience for you**.

I feel like I've found a hidden treasure when it comes to the experience of natural childbirth. And instead of keeping this treasure hidden, I want to share it with you.

Don't Just Take it From Me

The information I share is backed up by **research** as well as **real-world** experiences. I posted two surveys to online natural childbirth message boards and received over 150 responses from women who have had natural births. This book includes inspiring personal stories and helpful advice from over 65 women who are just like you!

Who is This Book For?

This book is for you if:

** **You are a first-time mom or new to natural birth.** You have an interest in natural birth, but you also have questions and concerns, including, "How do I start preparing for a natural birth?" Bring your curiosity and your open mind; I will help you deepen your determination, answer the most common questions asked about natural birth, and open your eyes to how birth can actually be a wonderful experience. (Really, it can be.)

** **You want a natural birth and are looking for support and guidance.** Perhaps your care provider doesn't know how to support a woman through a natural birth. Perhaps you don't know anyone who has birthed naturally. Perhaps you want advice and inspiration from moms who have had natural births. I share my path to natural births, hoping that it can help you on your path.

** **You are just starting your research.** I share a lot of helpful information, but there are many other great books that I recommend also, many of which go into much greater detail. (If you have read ALL the natural birth books already, you are probably set.)

** **You want convenience.** You may not have time to spend hour after hour, day after day combing the internet for all the advice you can find. This book shares the five keys to a natural birth and the supporting tips, inspiring stories, and a guide to fully preparing your body, mind, and spirit for a natural birth.

** **You plan to birth in a freestanding birth center, your own home, or a hospital.** Most of the information I share will be useful in planning a natural birth regardless of where you choose to birth. Helping you find your courage is universal to birth location. Extra tips and stories from natural hospital births are included.

Why Do You Need This Book?

It isn't enough to simply say, "I'm going to try to go natural."

Paradox of Natural Birth: Just because it's natural doesn't mean you don't need to prepare for it.

Preparing for a natural birth involves much more than just figuring out how to manage the pain during labor. The mental preparation is one of the most important—and often overlooked—preparations you can make.

But Can I Really Have a Natural Birth?

Yes, you can!

"There are only choices, not predestined sorts of people." – *Seth Godin*

Birthing your baby naturally is a choice. Don't believe you aren't the sort of person who could birth naturally.

You can.

But What About the PAIN?

Good news! Women who are more **confident in their ability to cope with labor** experience **less pain during labor**. Your job is to increase your confidence and courage. And that's what this book is about.

In this book I share the path I took to achieve two natural births. This is what worked for me and I hope it helps you on your journey. Keep in mind that you may have different experiences, though, because *nature is unpredictable* and *our bodies are not machines*.

In the end I hope your experience is like mine in the following ways:

** You know your role is important.

** You feel confident in your knowledge to voice your opinions and desires.

** You feel nurtured and loved by your care provider, and trust them to help you achieve your desires.

** You know your voice will be respected and heard, and your wishes valued and honored.

** Any wavering in your confidence will be met with multiple offerings of support and reminders that you can do this.

Defining Natural Childbirth

There are many ways in which people use the word "natural" regarding birth. For example, some people use "natural birth" to describe a birth that was not a cesarean section, when "vaginal birth" would be more accurate.

For this book, when I talk about natural childbirth I refer to an unmedicated vaginal birth, which means receiving no analgesia or anesthesia of any kind during labor and/or birth. (Analgesic=loss of pain. Anesthetic=loss of feeling.)

PART 1: PRE-LABOR PREPARATION: THE FIVE KEYS TO NATURAL BIRTH

Hoping for a natural birth is not enough. Would you sign up to run a marathon and then not train for it, simply showing up on race day and hoping for the best? Surely not.

I have found, with myself and from talking to others, that the more a woman prepares for her natural birth during her pregnancy——the more educated she is about her body, the birthing process, and her role in it—— the more likely she is to have the natural birth of her dreams.

The knowledge you gain about the birthing process will give strength to your voice: to ask questions of your medical providers with confidence.

You will learn the importance of **being vulnerable and surrendering completely** to the process of labor and birth.

You will learn the importance of having a **positive mental attitude**, reducing and removing any mental preoccupations which impede the ability to submit to labor.

You will learn to seek out excellent support.

You will learn to be patient; to have realistic expectations of the labor process.

It's true that it's important to learn *about* birth.

But it's also true that you *already know how to birth*.

Sharing Stories: Pre-Labor Preparation

"Pregnancy is beautifully designed to give a new mother the time to prepare for the birth. I worked hard during my pregnancy to make my natural birth a success." – Leah

"[Most helpful during labor was] the preparation I had done BEFORE labor started!" – Michelle

"[Most helpful during labor was] my training and preparation." – Cathryn

CHAPTER 1
FROM DESIRE TO DETERMINATION

"Determine that the thing can and shall be done, and then we shall find the way." – Abraham Lincoln

By purchasing this book, you already have a desire for a natural childbirth. You will also need **determination and commitment**.

Determination is born from a deep, internal conviction. No external challenges—or challengers—can sway you once you have made your decision.

There is great time and energy commitment in preparing for a natural birth. Determination will carry you through it.

As with anything worth achieving, your road to having a natural birth may have obstacles along the way. Determination is what will get you through those obstacles.

There is great physical, mental, and emotional work that is required during labor and birth. Determination will carry you through it.

Determine That Natural Childbirth Can Be Done

For thousands of years women have been having natural births—except they were just called "births." In the absence of a medicalized pain-free birth, there was nothing with which to compare birth in order for it to earn the distinction of "natural."

Since pain relief during labor and birth became more common during the 19th and 20th centuries, we have become removed from knowing birth as natural and from believing that we CAN birth a baby naturally, without pain medication.

But we still can.

And we still do.

Even though the percentage is small, there are many natural births in the United States each year. Let's look at some numbers for 2013:

** 3,876,042 hospital births

** 36,080 home births

** 16,913 freestanding birth center births

In one survey, 17% of women who birthed at hospitals reported using no pain medication during labor. If we extrapolate that statistic to the number of hospital births, that would indicate that there were approximately 658,927 natural births in hospitals. Combining the natural hospitals births with the home births and birth center births would indicate that there were approximately 711,920 natural births in the United States in 2013 (which is about 18% of all U.S. births).

Almost 1 in 5 U.S. births are natural!

It can be done. It is being done.

And you can do it too!

How Do You Become Determined?

Developing your determination will be different for every individual. I recommend taking some time for self-reflection, perhaps by meditating or journaling. These practices offer great opportunity to hear your own voice and to allow your deeper truths to come through. You can explore your inner voice on the following questions:

** Why do you want to have a natural birth?

** What reason is more important than any pain or challenge you may encounter?

Keep these questions in the back of your mind as you read this book. Once your knowledge about natural childbirth grows, your determination to stick with it will grow also.

Sharing Stories: Determination

Many moms shared with me what solidified their determination to have a natural birth. While the details of each mom's determination were different, there were several high-level reasons that were common:

** They believed it was healthiest for baby and mom.

** They believed their bodies were meant to birth naturally.

** They grew up in an atmosphere where natural birth was the norm.

** They wanted to feel everything and be part of the entire birthing experience.

** They wanted a challenge, or wanted to prove to themselves they could do it.

** They wanted to feel in control of their body.

** They did not like a previous medicalized birth.

** They wanted to avoid unnecessary interventions, concerned by their risks.

** They wanted a smoother recovery.

** They had a fear of needles and, therefore, epidurals.

** They wanted to avoid a cesarean section.

"I had an epidural with my son and felt like I missed something by not feeling everything. This piqued my interest. But the idea of a smoother recovery and better for my baby solidified my decision." – Talitha

"I did not like my experience with my previous medicated birth. I felt weak and out of it. I wasn't able to enjoy the moment that my child entered the world because I was so 'drugged up' so to speak." – Amber

"I wanted to feel well after delivery. With #1 I had an epidural; I didn't like that I couldn't move around after he was born. [With] #2 I had an IV pain drug; I felt high for hours after delivery. I was too nervous to nurse without someone standing beside me in case I would drop her, I felt that out-of-it." – Jen

"I have been sober for six years but was an active alcoholic and drug addict for almost a decade. Achieving a natural childbirth was about proving to myself that I took my sobriety seriously, that I was strong and capable, that I cared more about my baby than I did about my comfort." – Dana

"Once I started researching the effects of pain meds and interventions on babies and mothers I was sold on going all natural. I wanted my baby to have the best possible start, and coming into the world on her own schedule, alert and having the best chance to breastfeed successfully all became my vision for her birth." – Angela

"Originally, I just wanted to avoid having a needle placed in my spine. It just sounded so risky to me. However, in preparing for my natural birth I learned about all of the beautiful benefits to baby, and I became determined. I wanted my baby to have the best possible start, like any mom, so I followed my heart." – Kali

"I did not want any unnecessary interventions, and wanted to be coherent and in control. To be able to move around, and to navigate the process rather than be someone else's patient. I've seen both kinds of births and the natural birth felt more right and was the right method to bring my child into the world." – Courtney

Inspiration From Those Who Birthed Before Us: Shaping Our Determination

Stories connect us. When you hear how other women felt about their natural births, you can picture yourself birthing naturally as well. You can gain inspiration and determination from hearing other women's natural birth stories. There is something inspiring when we find out other women can and do birth their babies naturally, especially now that we have a choice about experiencing labor pain.

Looking to the Past

Hundreds of years ago women didn't have a choice but to endure the pain that comes with childbirth, but they found ways to cope. Social birth was the norm; women gathered together to help throughout the labor, birth, and beyond.

Thinking of the past and reflecting on the natural ability of women's bodies to birth babies may inspire you. Perhaps it will inspire you to find natural ways to cope with labor pain, such as being surrounded by continuous, loving support.

Looking to the Present

If you have a close friend or family member who has had a natural childbirth, you may have already found something inspiring in her story. Because we have a choice about whether to experience labor pain or not, these stories may simultaneously strike us curious and inspired as we ask: *why would anyone today choose to birth a baby without pain medication?*

Sharing Stories: Inspiration from Past and Present

"My mother had natural births, my sister had natural births, and I knew I could do it too." – Tabitha

"My grandma and my mom all birthed naturally and unmedicated, so they were my inspiration." – Annette

"The women in my life mostly presented birth as 'no big deal,' and natural birth as the default barring complications." – Sara

"I knew my cousin had home births and I loved hearing her experiences." – Jessica

"Having a natural birth was important to me because my mother had her children naturally, and I had grown up hearing how it gives babies the best start in life." – Kristen

"My family has all had natural childbirths (even with my dad being a doc)!" – Stacy

"My mother had three natural births and she spoke about them and the process of birth with such an awe." – Nadine

What do women who have had natural births today have to say about their experiences?

** Felt great immediately after birth, able to get up and walk right away.

** Pain gone right away, shut off like a switch.

** Recovered quickly.

** It was hard but doable. Not as bad as they thought it would be.

** It is pain easily forgotten (within hours).

** Wanted to have a natural birth again.

How did they feel after their natural birth(s)?

Along with feelings of being tired, sore, relieved, and hungry, moms shared many positive feelings, too:

** Amazing, wonderful, fantastic, awesome, euphoric, excited, fabulous.

** Content, comfortable, fully engaged, loving, grateful.

** Strong, empowered, like they could do anything.

** Proud, accomplished, confident, complete.

** Energized, alive, high on endorphins.

** ***Beautiful.***

Even when the births didn't go as expected, were harder, longer, or more difficult, upon reflection they realized the experience was wonderful.

Sharing Stories: Feelings After Natural Birth

"A high on life I never knew existed." – Nadine

"I love my body more than ever now that I know what it's really capable of. I feel like a superwoman." – Andrea

"I never had good self-esteem until I had my home birth. After that, I looked at myself in a different light. I was proud of myself and my body. It was amazing." – Amy

"Happy that I gave my baby such a wonderful gift. I know I got her life and our relationship off to a wonderful start." – Marissa

"I loved feeling every move of the baby and how my body responded." – Kayla

"I felt the happiest I have ever felt in my life, and overwhelmed with love. I felt proud that I had grown an actual human being inside of me and then opened myself up and pushed her out as well. I felt like an accomplished warrior." – Chenae

"Amazing. It was by far better than a hospital recovery and I felt so much better after having my second baby and it took less time on recovery overall. It was just powerful how my second daughter got here and how great I felt after having her." – Alex

"I felt wonderful and fully engaged with my baby girl. It was the best experience ever!" – Amber

"Fantastic, I felt empowered and calm, like I had just accomplished something amazing. Oh, and tired." – Laurel

"To be honest, at first I felt like I could never do it again. ... Now I look back on my experience and I am proud of myself. I feel more prepared to go natural again." – Tabitha

"[I felt] tired and a little shocked and proud of myself and euphoric, all at once." – Delilah

"Yes I had pain and I was tired, but I had this wonderful sense of accomplishment. It was also very special for my relationship with my husband; it was something we both had to go through together." – Erin

"It was really an intense experience, but the most wonderful thing I have ever been a part of." – Samantha

Magic of Natural Birth: It's Not About the Pain

It is interesting to note that many women chose to pursue a natural birth for its perceived physical benefits (healthier for mom and baby, better establish breastfeeding, quicker recovery).

But the surprise comes after the natural birth has happened, when you realize all the emotional benefits as well (empowered, strong, accomplished, beautiful).

You come away from the experience changed in ways you didn't expect.

And that is the magic of natural birth for me.

Divine Inspiration

"Birthing is the most profound initiation to spirituality a woman can have." – *Robin Lim*

I believe that in birth there is a spiritual connection to the divine. It is a chance to use our unique ability to bring life into this world, to bring forth something from nothing, to assist in a true miracle.

During labor and birth you will need to surrender to the process and accept what is happening. You need to have faith: faith in your body, faith in your baby, faith in the process.

Amazing. Awesome. Beautiful. Empowering.

I try to describe my natural births with these adjectives, but somehow they don't really do the experience justice. Natural birth is a deeply personal experience, not something that can easily (or correctly) be described with words.

Sounds like the divine to me.

We Shall Find the Way

I want to help you view labor not as an ordeal you must endure, but rather an important job that only you can do. You are important. The work you are doing is important.

** Stay true to your desire.

** The fundamentals of determination and commitment must be your fuel.

** Inspiration from others who have birthed naturally—past and present—will help you see that you can do it too!

** The work is great. The rewards are greater.

I'm not saying it's going to be easy.

I'm saying it's going to be worth it.

"Courage is not the absence of fear, but rather the judgment that something else is more important than one's fear." – *Ambrose Redmoon*

CHAPTER 2
BE INFORMED, BE INSPIRED

"Nothing in life is to be feared. It is only to be understood." – Marie Curie

Fear exists in the unknown.

Many women today are afraid of labor and birth, possibly because they don't know exactly what happens when a human female labors and births a baby.

I would add that with labor and birth there is also a fear of the "known," quotes intentional. For what many women "know" about labor and birth—what they fear about it and what they believe to be true—isn't the entire truth. Women today are getting their "knowledge" about labor and birth through dramatic birth scenes on TV and negative birth experiences shared by other women.

It was different over a hundred years ago when social birth was the norm. Women gained an intimate and accurate knowledge of the labor and birth process.

Times have changed and birth is no longer a social event shared with other women. As such, we have lost touch with truly knowing (and appreciating) the natural process of labor and birth. Most of us have never helped another woman through her labor or seen a baby being born in person.

In the absence of first-hand knowledge, we have to learn about the natural birth process on our own in other ways.

Informed About Birth: Inspired to Find Your Confidence

"When you change the way you view birth, the way you birth will change." – Marie Mongan

Your attitudes and feelings about childbirth are important factors related to birth outcome. According to one study, women who were **least afraid of childbirth** and **viewed it as a natural process** had the highest rate of unassisted vaginal births.

Once you gain knowledge about the physiological processes that work together during labor and birth (and the interventions that can lead a normal birth astray), you will start to view birth as normal and you will know that a woman's body was designed to birth a baby.

Normalizing birth reduces fears.

Once birth is viewed as normal, your fears will be reduced or even eliminated. And what will replace your fear is confidence.

** Confidence in your body's ability to birth a baby.

** Confidence in your baby to know how to be born.

** Confidence in yourself to figure out a way to handle it.

By normalizing birth, it will be easier to accept a drug-free birth for yourself. You will know that whatever your body is doing and what you are feeling is a NORMAL part of the process. There is no need to fight against or medicate normal.

Our culture tends to view pregnancy and childbirth as a disease or sickness and something from which you need rescuing. To start normalizing birth, immerse yourself in a world of books that view birth as normal.

Information and Inspiration from Books

With each book read, your knowledge about natural birth will grow and with it your courage and confidence. I recommend reading:

** Books about the physiological process of natural, healthy pregnancy and childbirth

** Books about all your birth choices

** Natural birth stories, so you can see the many ways natural birth can happen

** About how midwives, who are experts in natural childbirth, handle pregnancy and childbirth (this is good information to know even if you plan to birth in a hospital with an obstetrician)

Here is a list of books I've read and would recommend for the top of your reading list:

** **The Thinking Woman's Guide to a Better Birth**, by Henci Goer: This is the first book I recommend to anyone who is pregnant, whether they want to have a natural childbirth or not. It provides scientific research on many birth choices, such as obstetrical procedures and interventions, so the reader can make informed decisions about her maternity care and birth.

** **Ina May's Guide to Childbirth**, by Ina May Gaskin: Written by a midwife, this book shares many inspirational birth stories from her clients as well as information about how to avoid many standard medical interventions.

** **Pregnancy, Childbirth, and the Newborn**, by Penny Simkin: This book contains wonderful explanations of everything you need to know about pregnancy and natural childbirth.

** **The Official Lamaze Guide: Giving Birth with Confidence (2nd edition)**, by Judith Lothian and Charlotte De Vries. This easy-to-read book provides information about how pregnancy and birth progress naturally, medical evidence for help in making informed decisions, as well as steps to take for relieving fear and managing pain during labor.

** **Natural Hospital Birth: The Best of Both Worlds**, by Cynthia Gabriel. This book, written by a doula, shares practical tips for achieving a natural birth in a hospital. Included is information about avoiding unnecessary interventions, how to talk with hospital staff, and natural birth stories.

** **Birth Matters: A Midwife's Manifesta**, by Ina May Gaskin. In this book, midwife Ina May Gaskin asserts that the way in which women become mothers is a women's rights issue. She shows how to trust women and value birth.

** **Baby Catcher: Chronicles of a Modern Midwife**, by Peggy Vincent: This midwife chronicles her life as a baby catcher. Reading about how she responded to births, both routine and emergency, really helped me relax and trust birth, trust myself, and trust my midwife.

There are many more books you can read, which are listed in the *Recommended Resources* appendix.

Information and Inspiration from Movies

In addition to reading about natural birth, there are also a few movies you can watch to inform and inspire you.

** **The Business of Being Born:** One of the most well-known documentaries on exploring the current system of maternity care in America, it follows the story of Ricki Lake's second pregnancy and her preparation for an unmedicated home birth. (thebusinessofbeingborn.com)

** **More Business of Being Born:** Also from Ricki Lake and Abby Epstein, this four-part DVD series continues their exploration of the modern maternity care system, offering a look at birthing options as well as sharing celebrity birth stories. (thebusinessofbeingborn.com)

** **Pregnant in America:** Documentary which follows a pregnant couple who decide to give birth outside the hospital system. They travel the country investigating American maternity care. You can watch this documentary on Hulu. (hulu.com/watch/235715)

** **Birth Story: Ina May Gaskin and the Farm Midwives:** This documentary detailing the beginning of midwife Ina May Gaskin's start in midwifery the subsequent opening of The Farm, which offers a different model of care for pregnant women that changed how many approached childbirth. It contains some birth videos from the midwives' archive collection that show childbirth in a way most people have never seen it. (birthstorymovie.com/the-film)

** **Orgasmic Birth:** Documentary featuring seven women and their partners who show the emotional, spiritual, and physical aspects that birth can bring. (orgasmicbirth.com)

** **It's My Body, My Baby, My Birth:** An educational childbirth film that tells the story of seven women and their journeys to natural childbirth. (itsmybodymybabymybirth.com/Home.html)

Inspiration from Birth Videos

Many women post videos of their natural birth online on YouTube. By watching these videos, you can see how natural births happen in many different ways. To narrow your search, you can look for videos that will be similar to where or how you may want to birth such as "natural home birth" or "natural hospital birth" or "Hypnobabies natural birth," etc.

Your inspiration and confidence will grow each time you watch a natural birth.

Sharing Stories: Information Brings Confidence

"I read a lot during my pregnancy and the statistics associated with childbirth interventions concerned me. I decided I would learn everything I could about natural childbirth and work towards trusting my body to do what it was designed to do. I read several books on midwifery that made me believe I could actually do this!" – Bonnie

"I spent a massive amount of time reading books, scouring the web for anything that may help me get the birth I was envisioning, watching birth videos, reading positive birth stories and affirmations all helped me to feel confident heading into labor." – Angela

"[Most helpful during pregnancy was] becoming informed about what's the range of normal and what my medical and other options are, pros and cons of everything." – Jamie

Informed About Interventions: Inspired to Find Your Choice and Your Voice

While beneficial when complications arise, many common medical interventions are used routinely when they are not truly needed.

Unnecessary medical interventions used during labor and childbirth can have unintended effects because they interfere with the normal physiology of labor and birth. Often these effects are new problems that are treated with further intervention, which may create more problems. This chain of events, known as the "cascade of interventions," can change the course of a woman's labor.

Knowledge is key in making informed decisions regarding the many childbirth options available.

Any intervention carries risk, and before you decide to choose (or accept) one of the common obstetrical procedures performed during labor and birth, you and your care provider need to have a discussion to determine the risks versus the benefits for your situation.

Common Medical Interventions

This list is an introduction to common medical interventions and how they affect normal labor. I **recommend more in-depth research from evidence-based resources**. You will then be able to engage in informed discussions with your caregivers.

** **Induction:** Labors induced or augmented with synthetic oxytocin (Pitocin) are different than labors that start naturally. Synthetic oxytocin can interfere with the mother's natural hormones during labor, causing contractions that are longer, stronger, and closer together. This can be harder on the baby than natural contractions. If the baby can't tolerate the contractions, it may lead to a now-necessary cesarean. Induction of labor usually involves an IV line, continuous electronic fetal monitoring (EFM), restriction of movement, and restriction of eating and drinking. Women are more likely to request an epidural during induced labors.

Be aware that some providers use misoprostol (Cytotec) for induction and cervical ripening even though it has not been approved by the FDA for this purpose. Once started, its effects cannot be stopped. It can have serious side effects, such as uterine hyperstimulation.

Some inductions are medically necessary but many inductions are due to reasons of convenience or other non-medical rationale, such as the baby is full term, wanting to be done with the pregnancy, or wanting to control timing. Sometimes a provider's concern about the size of the baby leads mothers to choose induction, a practice that is not supported by best evidence.

Be patient; your baby knows how and when to be born. Research natural ways to start labor (verify with your care provider before using) such as long walks, nipple stimulation, acupuncture, acupressure points, using herbs, and castor oil. Eating dates during the last month of pregnancy may help reduce the need for induction or augmentation of labor.

** **Artificial Rupture of Membranes:** An intact amniotic sac protects the baby and your uterus from germs. Due to an increased risk of infection from repeated vaginal exams, once your bag of water is broken your care provider will probably want your baby to be born within a certain amount of time (usually 12-24 hours). This can increase the use of other interventions such as Pitocin, EFM, IV, restriction of movement, and may possibly lead to a cesarean.

Research other ways to get a slow labor moving, such as movement and hydration.

** **Routine Continuous Electronic Fetal Monitoring (EFM):** Compared with intermittent auscultation, routine continuous EFM increases the risk of cesarean for mothers while having no significant improvement in the overall perinatal death rate. The American Congress of Obstetricians and Gynecologists (ACOG) says either intermittent listening with a stethoscope or continuous EFM may be used for women who don't have complications. When connected to an EFM machine you will lose mobility, possibly hindering your ability to cope with contractions.

Ask your caregiver to perform intermittent fetal monitoring using a hand-held Doppler or fetoscope if there are no risk factors that would indicate the need for continuous EFM.

** **Routine Intravenous (IV) Fluids:** Routine IV use restricts movement, may lead to fluid overload (which can lead to problems with breastfeeding, baby losing weight, baby with jaundice, fluid in mom's and/or baby's lungs), and may contribute to low blood sugar in newborns. The American Society of Anesthesiologists (ASA) and the ACOG recommend allowing low-risk laboring women to drink clear liquids.

To stay hydrated and keep up strength, drink liquids as you feel like it. In the absence of certain interventions like inductions or epidurals, you should be able to decline a routine IV. But if your hospital requires one you could ask for a saline lock as a compromise. If the IV is only needed at certain times (for medications), ask to have it disconnected between doses.

** **Epidural:** Epidurals interfere with birth hormones, slowing labor and making pushing more difficult; all of which can lead to increased use of vaginal instruments (forceps or vacuum-extraction), episiotomy, and a cesarean. Epidural drugs do reach the baby and can cause disturbances of the fetal heart rate and other adverse effects. Initiation of breastfeeding can be more difficult after epidural use. Epidurals keep a woman confined to bed for labor and birth. If you have an epidural you will need an IV, continuous EFM, and a bladder catheter.

** **Restriction of Movement:** The use of interventions can require restriction of movement, as mentioned above. But movement is an important part of labor and birth. Nature cues you with labor pain so you can move and adjust accordingly to help baby rotate, descend, and find the optimal position for birth. Movement such as walking and changing positions can relieve pain and shorten labor. Walking in early labor can reduce the chances of a cesarean.

In the absence of a complication walk and move as you feel, perhaps by laboring at home as long as you can. Also, choose a birth site that allows freedom of movement during labor and birth.

Sharing Stories: Informed About Interventions

During labor, a doctor mentioned using a certain intervention to my friend Juliana and her husband. Instead of just accepting the recommendation they kindly asked the doctor, "Is this medically necessary or is it just to speed things up? Because we are fine with waiting." The intervention was not medically necessary so they declined it, and went on to have their natural birth. Both knowing their options and being willing speak up in kind conversation with the doctors was valuable in ensuring their natural hospital birth.

"You need to be educated on pregnancy/birth and be prepared for 'detours.' Not every birth is problem-free and you need to know your options in case your labor takes an unexpected turn." – Michelle

Information Can Inspire

By immersing yourself in knowledge about natural birth, as well as interventions that can hinder natural birth, the following will happen:

** You will view birth as a normal process, one that you are innately capable of doing.

** Your fears will be reduced and your confidence will grow.

** Your resolve to avoid unnecessary interventions will be strengthened.

** You will be able to engage in informed discussions with your caregivers.

** You will be empowered by taking part in creating options that fit you.

If information overload sets in, come back to this thought: **you already know how to birth**.

"Giving birth should be your greatest achievement, not your greatest fear." – Jane Weideman

CHAPTER 3
FIND YOUR SUPPORT AND YOUR STRENGTH
WILL FOLLOW

"...Respecting the woman as an important and valuable human being and making certain that the woman's experience while giving birth is fulfilling and empowering is not just a nice extra, it is absolutely essential as it makes the woman strong and therefore makes society strong." – Marsden Wagner

As women, we intuitively know how to give birth. But that doesn't mean we don't need and deserve support. For a woman to have a natural childbirth she needs:
   ** A supportive caregiver
   ** A supportive birthing environment
   ** Supportive people around her, during pregnancy as well as during labor and birth

Importance of Choosing a Supportive Caregiver

"Women's strongest feelings [in terms of their birthings], positive and negative, focus on the way they were treated by their caregivers." – Annie Kennedy and Penny Simkin

The most important decision you will make during pregnancy is the choice of a caregiver and birth location; the two are often connected.

It's important to choose a caregiver for the right reasons. I caution against some of the common ways in which women today choose their caregiver, such as insurance coverage, convenience of location, and recommendations from friends (who may have wanted a different birth experience).

You want to have a high-quality relationship with your caregiver. In addition to finding a caregiver who is trained and competent, look for the following:

** Caregiver who follows evidence-based maternity care.

** Caregiver who uses shared decision-making processes.

** Caregiver who reaffirms a woman's natural ability to grow, nurture, and birth a baby.

** Caregiver with understanding that pregnancy and birth is not only a physical experience, but a mental, emotional, and spiritual one as well.

** Caregiver who fully supports you and your choice of natural birth.

Questions to Ask Your Caregiver

MotherFriendly.org offers a list of 10 questions to ask your caregiver/birth location to determine if they support the philosophy of mother-friendly care (motherfriendly.org/downloads). This list was created by the Coalition for Improving Maternity Services (CIMS). You can also read their list of 10 steps of Mother-Friendly care, as well as many other resource articles.

Options for Caregivers: Midwives

Midwives typically follow the midwifery model of care, which involves a focus on staying healthy and preventing problems. They view pregnancy and birth as normal physiological processes that require medical intervention only in special circumstances. Care during pregnancy and birth tends to be individualized. Practicing woman-centered maternity care, midwives tend to incorporate shared decision-making. Also, language such as "midwives catch babies" and "the mother gives birth" is common.

With their focus on a holistic approach to pregnancy and birth, midwives will help you prepare physically as well as emotionally for your natural birth. Prenatal appointments can be 30 minutes long.

Midwives deal with normal, low-risk pregnancies; complications are rare. The majority of pregnancies (70-80%) are considered low-risk.

A midwife's knowledge and support can help prevent problems. However, midwives are well-trained to recognize signs of complications developing and are able to handle most of them. She can also transfer your care to a physician backup if the need arises.

Many midwives provide continuous support throughout labor and birth. They often encourage and provide support for breastfeeding.

There are different types of midwives practicing in various settings.

** **Certified Nurse Midwives (CNMs)** are registered nurses who have completed additional postgraduate training from a nurse-midwifery education program accredited by the American College of Nurse-Midwives (ACNM). Most CNMs attend births in hospitals, but they also attend births in freestanding birth centers and in private homes.

 ** **Certified Professional Midwives (CPMs)** have trained in midwifery (but are not registered nurses) and are certified by the North American Registry of Midwives (NARM). Most CPMs attend births in private homes or in freestanding birth centers; they usually do not practice in hospitals.

 ** **Certified Midwife (CM)** is a new credential from the ACNM that does not require a nursing degree but is otherwise similar to the CNM credential.

How To Know if You are Considered Low-Risk

The criteria for accepting a client varies between midwives. The best way to determine if you are considered low-risk is to meet with a midwife in your area for a consultation. You can discuss your health and share any concerns or health-related questions you have. They can share their criteria and help you determine if midwifery care would be a good fit for you.

Sharing My Story

 My prenatal appointments with my midwife were 30 minutes long and very relaxed and conversational. I weighed myself and tested my own urine. A good majority of the appointment was spent talking about any questions or concerns I had. The rest of the time was spent seeing to the physical aspects, such as listening to the baby's heartbeat, checking my blood pressure, measuring my fundal height, and palpating my abdomen.

Options for Caregivers: Physicians

Physicians typically follow the medical model of maternity care, which involves a focus on diagnosing and managing problems and complications. They may tend to have a more narrow range of normal regarding pregnancy and birth, which leads to more dependence on technology; the use of interventions is common during labor. Care during pregnancy and birth tends to be routine for everyone.

 As part of provider-centered care, physicians are usually the decision-makers during pregnancy and birth. Also, language such as "doctors deliver babies" is common.

 With their focus on physical problems they may give less attention to emotional concerns.

 Women with serious health problems, risks for problems, or who develop complications will need the expertise of an obstetrician. However, since the majority of pregnancies are considered low-risk, an obstetrician may not have the most benefit.

 Physicians are usually not present during labor, but show up to catch the baby toward the end. Most physicians attend births in hospitals.

How Do You Know if Your Doctor is Supportive of Natural Birth?

I recommend discussing your plans for natural childbirth with your doctor during your prenatal visits. Hearing any of the following responses from your doctor regarding your natural birth plans would be considered a red flag regarding their support:

** "Don't be a hero."
** "You might change your mind."
** "I'm no fan of pain."
** "It's not a contest."
** "There's no medal for doing it without drugs."
** "Most of my patients choose an epidural, but I suppose you can try to go natural if you want."

Sharing Stories: Finding the Right Caregiver

"I switched doctors six months into my pregnancy after I had a more detailed talk with her about the type of birth we wanted. She did not see eye to eye with us. It was one of the best decisions we made, to change practices to someone who was much more aligned with our vision." – Samantha

"[Most helpful during pregnancy was] choosing an OB that was 110% supportive of a natural birth, believing that my body was designed to give birth, and that I could do it." – Dianthe

"Find a provider who supports you and with experience in natural birth." – Kimberly

"Have trust in your care providers/attendants and get to know the setting you'll be giving birth in, if you can. ... If you trust your care providers, you'll have an easier time letting go." – Margaret

"[Most helpful during labor was] staying calm, having a great support person with me, and my doctor really wanting to help me go natural." – Monique

Most Supportive Environment for Natural Childbirth: Where Do You Feel Safe and Supported?

To have a natural childbirth, choose a birth environment where you feel the safest and most confident. In order to relax and surrender to the process, you need to be where you feel the safest. What it means to feel safe and supported during labor and birth will vary from woman to woman.

** **Emotional safety:** To feel safe during childbirth, women need to feel respected. This respect can be a respect for their desires and for their capability to birth. They want to be consulted as an important part of the birthing process. They need their birthing space to be regarded as sacred.

** **Physical safety:** To feel safe during childbirth, women need to feel their physical needs are being taken care of. They need to feel they are cared for by experienced professionals who know what to do in case of emergency.

The location of supportive environments for natural childbirth could be home, birth center, or hospital.

Sharing Stories: Create a Safe Environment

"Create an atmosphere that supports what you want. I felt safest in a hospital atmosphere with a midwife attending me." – Bonnie

"Choose a birth place/care provider which fit well with what you want and where/with whom you feel the safest and most relaxed." – Delilah

"I had an unnecessary induction with my first. It was traumatic and we both walked away with minor injuries. After that I researched my options and found homebirth to be safest for our family." – Fonda

Birth Center and Home Birth: The Natural Place for Natural Birth

Birthing at home or in a freestanding birth center are safe, valid, and excellent options for those planning a natural childbirth. If you choose your home or a freestanding birth center for your birth, you will most likely be under the care of a midwife.

** Freestanding birth centers are usually staffed by Certified Nurse Midwives (CNMs) who provide all prenatal care and attend the birth of your baby at the birth center or maybe even at your home.

** Home births are usually attended by Certified Professional Midwives (CPMs) who provide all prenatal care and attend the birth of your baby at your home. Some CNMs attend home births as well.

Midwives who attend births at a freestanding birth center or at home do not have access to epidurals. This is good news for your natural birth goal!

Choosing a birth center or home birth with a midwife attending is a good option for:

** Women with healthy, low-risk pregnancies

** Women who are highly motivated to participate in their prenatal care

** Women who feel safe and confident in those environments

Sharing Stories: Birth Center

"I think also being in a birthing center where no one even questioned my ability to handle childbirth or even offer pain meds also helped." – Adriana

Natural Childbirth in a Hospital

Natural childbirth in a hospital is possible. However, it will be more difficult to achieve and will require more determination, support, and preparation due to the easy access to epidurals and the experience, attitudes, and policies of the hospital and its staff, which lean toward the medicalization of birth. If you are surrounded by people who don't support and encourage your natural childbirth choice (including your doctor and nurses), you might be talked into something you don't want. And in the middle of labor all your wishes for a natural birth can go out the window if you know an epidural is in the building.

Support for natural childbirth in a hospital setting will vary among hospitals and among doctors and staff. Some nurses and doctors may not be supportive of a patient who wants a natural childbirth. This will deviate from their standard procedures. On the flip side, some nurses are thrilled to help support a mama through a natural birth. They feel important and needed during this special time.

Some hospitals employ CNMs, which might be a good choice for a care provider if you choose birth in a hospital setting. A hospital-based midwife will most likely support you in your natural childbirth goal, although they may still be bound by certain hospital regulations or restrictions.

Some hospitals have policies that are not supportive of natural childbirth, such as forbidding one or more of the following: birth balls, labor tubs, showers, walking, and doulas.

Since your desire for natural childbirth is not common in a hospital setting, you will have to make your wishes known and advocate for them. I recommend your partner help advocate for you since you will be deeply focused on the work of labor.

Unfortunately you probably won't be able to know before labor starts who will be your support staff at the hospital. But you can find out the policies and procedures in your hospital ahead of time. You can ask your doctor about their experiences with natural birth in your hospital. Understanding your options in a hospital setting can help you create a safe birthing space. And if need be, you can always find a different birthing location more in line with your wishes.

Sharing Stories: Varying Support From Hospital Staff

"I had a doctor and nurses looking at me like 'Yeah sure...a natural childbirth' and they would constantly ask me if I was ready for an epidural. I would just tell them to give me some space and [then I would] look at my husband. Don't listen to anyone who says you can't do it." – Kayla

"I got to the hospital at 8cm and due to a posterior baby stayed there for three hours. The nurse stayed by my side and didn't 'permit' me to get hysterical or too emotional. Her stoic nature was what I needed to keep as calm as possible." – Mirja

"My husband, midwife, nurses, and hospital were all helpful in attaining my natural birth. Everyone was supportive and kept me on track at times when I thought I couldn't do it." – Tabitha

"We were at a hospital that was known for being supportive of natural childbirth so the staff there was supportive too." – Samantha

"[Most helpful during labor was] staying home as long as possible in my one hospital birth and my husband advocating for me while we were there. Staying out of the hospital

altogether in my others." – Jamie

"Choose a provider who shares your passion for a natural birth. Choose a facility that also values moms and babies. My hospital birth was fantastic that way. I only had to decline the anesthesiologist once. Then the nurses were very supportive and encouraging....Choosing a compatible provider and location are super important." – Jessica

Surround Yourself With Supportive People During Pregnancy

As a woman planning a natural childbirth, you understand that the bulk of the work of bringing your baby into the world is yours. But that doesn't mean you don't need – and deserve – support along the way.

Having a supportive partner is imperative for natural childbirth. Your partner should play an active role in the pre-labor preparation, attending natural childbirth classes as well as reading literature on natural birth. Remind your partner that he or she is your best support.

During pregnancy, only surround yourself with people who believe you can do it and who support your belief in yourself. If friends or family aren't supportive of your goal, politely remind them that you believe in yourself, your body, and your baby, and you do not wish to hear any negative comments.

The same goes with anyone who tries to share their negative birth story with you or tries to dissuade you from pursuing a natural birth.

"Never let the noise of other people's opinions drown out your own inner voice." – Steve Jobs

Find Your Natural Birth Tribe

I recommend finding a group of like-minded women for support during pregnancy, women who have birthed naturally or are planning to birth naturally, women supporting other women in their natural birth journey. Whether in person or online, having a supportive group can help you find and keep your strength. Look for:
   ** Any family or friends who have had a natural childbirth.
   ** People you meet in your natural childbirth class.
   ** Online message boards or groups, such as Mothering.com and BabyCenter.com's Natural Unmedicated Childbirth forum.
Sisterhood is powerful. In tribes there is strength.

Sharing Stories: Connecting With a Natural Birth Tribe

"I would ask other women about their experiences, and for the most part, if not all, they were the 'horror' stories of how painful [it was] and that I should get an epidural or just have a c-section. The interesting thing was that no one shared tips on how to cope with the contractions or shared a positive experience. ... I followed the [BabyCenter.com] forum called "Natural Unmedicated Childbirth". The positive stories that other women

posted really helped me with my first childbirth." – *Julia*

"Talk with women who have had a natural birth. The connection with a community of women will help you feel strong and prepared." – *Leah*

Surround Yourself With Supportive People During Labor

During labor and birth, only surround yourself with people who will be a reassuring presence, who give you confidence, and who fully support your choices in labor. Your birth support team is there to serve you. This may mean simply your partner and your caregiver. Or it may include other women you are close to and want present, such as a sister, friend, or mother.

This is your birth and you need to create your own comfortable environment of support. Be selective about who will be present and who will not, keeping in mind that you can relax and focus better if you don't feel observed or judged.

"Birth is not a party, like a wedding, where you have to worry about offending those who were not invited ... You should only invite people you trust, who approve of your birth plan, and who you don't mind seeing you naked." – *Ricki Lake and Abby Epstein*

Sharing Stories: Support During Labor

"Have a good, well-informed birth partner who knows you well and will accompany you through [labor and delivery]. There will be many times you may not think clearly so you want someone who will think clearly for you." – *Ashley*

"I also made my husband promise to stay strong and determined along with me. He has a hard time seeing me in pain so we talked about it ahead of time." – *Karen H.*

"The support from my husband was most helpful in attaining my natural birth. He encouraged me and was my advocate." – *Tabitha*

"My husband was the most helpful, he kept me focused and encouraged me constantly." – *Laurel*

"[Most helpful during labor was] the support of my husband and mother. My midwife was great." – *Cathryn*

"[Most helpful during labor was] my midwife. My husband. Confidence in myself, my body, and my decisions." – *Kelly*

Labor Support: Hire a Doula

Continuous emotional and physical support is key in having a natural birth. Your partner is your best labor support, but if you don't have a partner, if you are birthing in a hospital, or if you want more support I suggest hiring a doula (pronounced DOO-luh).

A doula is a person who provides continuous emotional support during labor and birth. Doulas do not perform medical tasks nor do they tell the doctor or nurses how to care for you. They can let you know what's going on with your labor and your options, remind you what you really want, and help you ask the right questions of your care providers according to your birthing preferences. They want to help you have a satisfying birth according to your wishes.

Having continuous support during labor and birth has many benefits, especially when the provider is not part of the hospital staff or the woman's social network such as with a doula. In addition to having slightly shorter labors, women with continuous support during labor were:

** Less likely to use any pain medication

** Less likely to have a cesarean section

** More likely to have spontaneous vaginal birth (no cesarean, vacuum-extraction, or forceps)

** Less likely to rate their childbirth experience negatively

Doulas are connected to natural birth. They observe you and will respond with the support you need at each stage of labor, which may include:

** Verbal support, such as encouragement and reassurance.

** Physical support, such as massage.

** Suggestions of comfort or coping techniques.

** Reminders of your wishes at key times, so you (or your partner) can advocate for yourself.

** Relieving your partner during a long labor.

Sharing Stories: Support From Doulas

"I was afraid I couldn't do it because so many people tell you that 'you don't need to be a superhero' or people say 'you are so small there is no way you can have a natural birth.' I did have a moment of panic the first time, but my doula got me up in a position where I felt powerful and it was fine after that." – Katie

"[Most helpful during labor was] my doula!" – Emily

"My doula was amazing. She was also our Bradley Childbirth class instructor, which really helped both me and my husband to relax, knowing we had that support and resource there with us." – Lauren

"[Most helpful during labor was] the double hip squeeze by my doula." – Dana

"If you're birthing in a hospital get a doula." – Fonda

"Our doula talked in depth with us about if we had concerns or fears." – Laurel

How to Find a Doula

To find a doula, ask for referrals from friends who have had great experiences, local midwives/birth centers, or childbirth educators.

You can also do a general search online or try one of these online directories of doulas:

** Childbirth and Postpartum Professional Association (CAPPA), icappa.net/search/custom.asp?id=438

** DONA International: Find a Doula, dona.org/mothers/find_a_doula.php

** Doula Match, doulamatch.net

** International Childbirth Education Association (ICEA), icea.org/content/member-directory

** List of volunteer doula programs, radicaldoula.com/becoming-a-doula/volunteer-programs

You may be able to find doulas in training who will attend your birth for no charge.

Keep in mind that each doula has a different practice style and different passion; not all doulas are equal. Interview doulas until you find good match. Don't feel bad if you don't hire a doula after she's interviewed with you. It's your birth and you need the support that is best suited for you.

In Support, You Find Strength

With support you can do this, and you will do this.

** Midwives are experts in natural birth and are a good option for low-risk women (which is most women). They nurture the family through a normal, physiological process.

** Physicians are experts in pathology and are a good option for high-risk women.

** Finding the right caregiver and birth location for **you and your birth vision** will bring you strength.

** Finding a natural birth tribe, like-minded women supporting each other through birth, can lead to a feeling of shared strength.

** Your partner is your best support during labor. Be sure he or she feels prepared to support you.

** Doulas provide excellent labor support and can especially be helpful for those birthing in a hospital or for those without a partner.

"The whole point of woman-centered birth is the knowledge that a woman is the birth power source. She may need, and deserve, help, but in essence, she always had, currently has, and will have the power." – Heather McCue

CHAPTER 4
NURTURE A BELIEF IN YOURSELF

"Whatever the mind can conceive and believe, it can achieve." – Napoleon Hill

The most important key to having a natural childbirth is the belief that you can do it.

Hundreds of years ago women didn't wonder if they could or could not have a natural childbirth. They knew they could because all women could.

Since pain medications have been used for birth, and especially since epidurals became so common, women have started doubting their ability to give birth without them. However:

As a woman, you've always had the ability to birth your baby naturally.

You have always had your own birth power, you just need to tap into it.

This doubt in your ability to work with your body during birth— expending great effort, reaching deeper inside yourself, transforming—is a new phenomenon. And you don't have to buy into it.

Forget the negative spin society plays on childbirth. You aren't crazy for choosing a natural birth. You don't have to be talented, special, athletic, or have a high pain tolerance (if there even is such a thing).

It matters not what anyone else thinks, says, or does; it only matters what *you* think, say, and do.

Your thoughts create your reality.

What reality are you creating for yourself? One filled with doubt and fear? Or one filled with confidence and courage?

You may need to change the paradigm of:
    ** How you view birth
    ** How you view your body
    ** How strong you believe yourself to be

There may be some barriers between you and a belief in your capability, such as a lack of knowledge about birth as normal and doubts about your role in the normal physiological process of birth.

We addressed increasing your knowledge about birth in chapter 2. Now, let's explore ways to help you **recognize your inherent capability to give birth**.

    ** Address and Clear Your Doubts and Fears
    ** Acknowledge Past Accomplishments
    ** Clear Your Mind, Create a Calm Place
    ** Create and State Daily Positive Affirmations
    ** Set Positive Birth Intentions
    ** Create a Positive Atmosphere

Address Your Doubts and Fears

Before they are addressed, any doubts or fears must first be identified. Here are a few questions for your personal reflection:

    ** What do you believe about childbirth?
    ** What is one of your worst fears about labor and birth?
    ** How do you feel about being "out of control" during labor?
    ** When thinking about pain during labor, what are you concerned about?
    ** When envisioning the physical process of giving birth, what are you concerned about?
    ** How do you currently feel about the support you are receiving from your partner? Your caregiver?
    ** How do you currently feel about your physical strength?
    ** How do you currently feel about your body? What do you like most about it? The least?

Sometimes just the simple act of reflecting on these areas and uncovering any doubts or fears will help lessen them.

Common Fears

Having some fears about pregnancy or birth is normal. Some common fears may include fear of pain, fear of losing control, fear of problems with the baby, and fear of your wishes not being respected, among others. I think they can fit under one big fear: the fear of the unknown.

Sharing Stories: Fears

"Don't be ashamed of any nerves or fear. Embrace them and plan on ways you can

work through those during the birth. Birthing is a very, very psychological process. Your emotions will influence how the experience goes. You'll go to a place you've never been before, where you need to be both strong and vulnerable at the same time." – Leah

"I had an epidural with my first and did not like it....I was afraid of the pain [of natural birth] but I was more afraid of the lack of control and feeling helpless that I got with the epidural." – Delilah

Clear Your Doubts and Fears: Sharing Some Stories

Many moms shared how they addressed any fears they had; the most common ways were:

** They discussed their fears with their caregivers.

** They talked with their partner or other close family or friends.

** They read positive natural birth stories.

** They did lots of research both online and reading books (especially those by Ina May Gaskin, and Childbirth Without Fear, by Grantly Dick-Read).

** They took natural birth classes (ones that specifically address fears are Hypnobabies and Birthing From Within).

** They repeated positive affirmations, visualizations, and meditation.

** They had faith, trust, and they prayed.

Sharing Stories: Addressing Fears

"I would get down to the root of the fear first and try to understand why I had that fear to begin with and then do research." – Adriana

"I addressed my fears by educating myself on the facts and reading encouraging natural childbirth stories from other women. I really came to believe that I could do this. I was also willing to acknowledge that if for some reason it became prudent (medically necessary) to change my mind during labor that was okay too." – Bonnie

"The best way [to address fears] is by hearing natural birth stories, reading lots of books about all the variety in normal births ... also discussing fears with my doula. Doing research regarding the negative effects of medical intervention in birth made me confident that my choices were scientifically backed and also worth it." – Jenny

"Honestly, my fears were mostly related to having to transfer to a facility for any reason and then having to FIGHT for what I knew baby and I needed, or what was best for us. I kept detailed, accurate records, kept myself healthy to minimize any possibility of risk, and just kept myself educated." - Bryn

"Throughout my pregnancy I would waiver between confident and nervous. When nervous I would read and talk to others. ... Connection with other women who had birthed naturally gave me the confidence I needed to face my fears." – Leah

"I followed the Birthing From Within method, which taught to address concerns through discussion with your partner, journaling, and birth art. I didn't have a lot of fears, though; I figured if women had been giving birth naturally since the beginning of humankind I could do it too!" – Kristen

"Finding support within the natural birthing community is key!" – Samantha

Discussing Fears with Caregiver

An ideal caregiver will provide a safe place for you to share any and all concerns you may have. They will do this by asking about your feelings toward pregnancy and birth, welcoming any of your questions about fears, and responding with empathy and compassion so you can feel confident.

Whether it's a concern about handling the pain of labor, the position of your baby, your caregiver not being on call when you go into labor, a worry about tearing, or a concern about pooping while birthing, they will be happy to help inform or reassure you.

If your caregiver does not spend time **each appointment** asking about your thoughts, feelings, and concerns, please bring up the questions yourself. It is so important to address and calm any fears you have and they have the ability to help.

Sharing My Story

During one early prenatal visit during my second pregnancy, I mentioned how I was afraid this birth wouldn't go as well as my first. My midwife was able to put words to a concern I wasn't even able to verbalize well myself, and sat by me offering tissues as I cried. She understood that since my first birth was perfectly smooth, my concern was "Can I have two wonderful births?"

After validating my concern, she was wonderful about reassuring me that yes, I could very well have two wonderful births. I am grateful she created a safe place for me to share concerns that were very real to me.

Sharing a Story: Discussing Fears with Caregivers

"I talked to my midwife about my concerns, listened to her based on her medical knowledge and experience, and then did my own research and made the best decision for myself and my family." – Michelle

Clear Your Doubts and Fears: Emotional Freedom Technique (EFT)

One technique that can be used to address fears is the Emotional Freedom Technique (EFT). A form of psychological acupressure, EFT involves tapping with the fingertips on certain meridians on the head and chest while thinking about a specific problem (such as a fear) and repeating positive affirmations.

While this type of technique may seem odd to many in the West, it is a method that has provided great results for many people and it is easy to do yourself. I did not use this method during my pregnancies, but have used it recently, and with good results.

There are three parts of EFT:

** Selecting an appropriate affirmation

** Tuning in to your problem by thinking about it

** While tapping, state the affirmations loudly with great enthusiasm

The statements you make while tapping may be said in two different ways:

** 1. **Stating the doubt or fear and then following it with love and acceptance of yourself.** For example: "Even though I have this fear of not being in total control of birth, I deeply and completely accept myself." or "Even though I doubt my ability to handle the pain, I deeply and completely love and accept myself."

** 2. **Say a positive statement that is the opposite of the doubt or fear.** For example: "I choose to feel confident in my body and my baby during labor and birth." or "Let it be easy to work with my body during labor." or "I choose to feel empowered during labor and birth."

For more information about the specific tapping points (photos and illustrations) as well as much more information to help get you started, check out this article on Mercola.com: eft.mercola.com.

Acknowledge Past Accomplishments: What Have You Done Already?

In preparing for a difficult challenge ahead, it's helpful to reflect on the difficult goals you have already accomplished in your life.

What are some difficult mental challenges you've overcome? Graduating college while holding down a job or two? Starting a new job or starting your own business? Solving a big problem at work? Learning a new skill, a musical instrument, or a foreign language?

What are some difficult physical challenges you've already accomplished? Perhaps you made the basketball team in college or completed a marathon?

If you take the time to reflect on your life so far, you will see the many ways you have successfully met physical or mental challenges.

You are stronger than you think you are.

Clear Your Mind, Create a Calm Place

Meditation and yoga are two excellent ways to calm your mind, which may also aid in reducing fears and leaving space for positive energy.

** **Meditation:** You can search for specific pregnancy meditations or do a simple meditation by closing your eyes and focusing on your breathing, letting your mind go completely clear. Start where you are, even if it means just five minutes at a time. I found this guided pregnancy meditation for releasing your fears on YouTube, which may be helpful. (youtube.com/watch?v=6Z4ARHBzX9Q)

** **Yoga:** Focusing on the breath while engaging in yoga exercises can bring both physical and mental balance. One type of yoga program specifically for pregnant women is Mamaste Yoga. (mamasteyoga.com)

Sharing Stories: Staying Calm

"[My yoga practice] showed me I could stay calm and collected with myself during strenuous times. If you hold a headstand for five minutes, you can't do a lot of other things besides learn to deal with yourself or freak out and leave the situation. Labor was a lot like standing on your head." – Kristen

"I used a guided relaxation fear release track found at www.thebirthyear.com." – Kali

"[Most helpful during pregnancy was] staying calm [and] really enjoying my pregnancy and the miracle that was happening." – Monique

Create and State Daily Positive Affirmations

"How often—even before we began—have we declared a task 'impossible'? And how often have we construed a picture of ourselves as being inadequate? … A great deal depends upon the thought patterns we choose and on the persistence with which we affirm them." – Piero Ferrucci

Affirmations are statements that, when repeated, can shape our thoughts and mindset. **Repeating positive affirmations daily** can help you change the way you think about many different aspects of pregnancy and birth, replacing fearful or negative thoughts with new positive ones.

Even if you don't 100% believe what you are affirming to yourself (yet) by saying the phrases, your subconscious will start to believe them.

** **Action:** Search through books and online to come up with a list of positive affirmations that affirm a safe, healthy, and comfortable pregnancy as well as confidence about your baby's health, timing of birth, and your ability to birth your baby naturally. Type these out on paper and **read them every day at the same time**, so it becomes a habit. You could even record yourself speaking the affirmations and listen to them.

Sharing My Story

I took the Hypnobabies home study course and it came with an audio track of "Joyful Pregnancy Affirmations" that **I listened to every day** usually on my drive home from work or on a walk. After listening to the affirmations daily for 10 weeks, the words became part of me. The affirmations played a huge role in growing my confidence, courage, and peace about the upcoming birth.

I credit these affirmations as a huge part of my empowering natural birth experience, and I highly recommend the entire Hypnobabies home study course.

Here are a few of my favorite Hypnobabies affirmations:

** Pregnancy is natural, normal, healthy, and safe for me and my baby.

** My baby is healthy and safe inside me now.

** I love my pregnant body and I accept it every day.
** My baby knows how and when to be born and I will be patient.
** I have faith that my baby will be born at the perfect time.
** Birth is a safe and wonderful experience for me.
** Birth is a safe and wonderful experience for my baby.
** My body is made to give birth easily and comfortably.
** I believe in my ability to give birth easily.
** I completely trust in my ability to birth my baby.

Birth Affirmations as Art

I recently came across a unique way to incorporate birth affirmations into your pregnancy: a birth affirmations coloring book! The Art of Birth (theartofbirth1.wix.com/theartofbirth) offers a coloring book with original hand-drawn birth images and affirmations. With a connection between birth and art, coloring these affirmation pages during pregnancy offers a chance to reflect and prepare for the birth. Once completed, you can hang them where you can see and read them every day, as well as during labor and birth.

Set Positive Birth Intentions: Visualize

Set the intention and expectation for your perfect natural birth.

Visualize your perfect, easy birth; when labor starts, how long it lasts, positions you want to labor in and birth in, who you want supporting you, how you feel, how you think, and the time of day. Picture everything you want your birth to be. Visualize it happening that way. Also visualize the steps you will take along the way to help achieve your natural birth. **Repeat this visualization often.**

Create a Positive Atmosphere

Creating a positive mindset for yourself is imperative for attaining your goal of natural childbirth. But since most of us don't live in a bubble, we will probably come in contact with others who do not share our focus on birth as normal and healthy.

Throughout your pregnancy you will also need to create a positive atmosphere around yourself, almost like a protective bubble. You need to protect your goal and dream and positive mindset from anything or anyone who may try to burst it, either intentionally or unintentionally.

To create a positive atmosphere I recommend the following:

** **Surround yourself with only positive natural birth stories.** Stories connect us. Every time you hear stories of other women being strong and capable in birth, you will associate yourself with being strong and capable as well. It will become easier to picture yourself having a positive natural childbirth.

Talk to women who have felt excited and empowered from their birth. Search for natural birth stories online or find them in books. Through reading and hearing many stories you will see all the many wonderful ways natural birth can happen, and you will see the wide range of normal.

Here are a couple resources for natural birth stories. Each site has stories sorted by category such as home births, hospital births, VBACs, etc.:

    ** Mama Birth (over 100 birth stories) (mamabirth.com/p/birth-stories.html)

    ** Giving Birth Naturally, givingbirthnaturally.com/birth-diaries.html

    ** Natural Childbirth Stories, naturalchildbirthstories.com

** ** Avert the negative birth stories.** Be warned that friends, family, or even strangers may share their scary/painful/disappointing birth story with you the moment you tell them your plans. Do not allow any bad stories into your consciousness.

My friend Carey Sue had an "exit strategy" she used when someone started telling her a disappointing birth story; it was a prepared sentence that would politely stop people from continuing. Perhaps something like "Thanks so much, but I only want to hear positive stories" will work.

** ** Surround yourself with only positive people.** Hopefully your friends and family are supportive of you and your goal of natural childbirth. However, you may need to keep your distance and reduce interaction with anyone who continually tries to rain on your parade, so to speak. Protecting your bubble of peace is very important in planning for a natural birth.

** ** Surround yourself with only positive messages about birth.** Stop watching those dramatic TV shows about birth; they will not help you prepare for natural childbirth. There are many inspiring books to read and videos to watch, as I noted earlier, which will actually help you remain positive and focused.

Sharing Stories: Importance of a Positive Atmosphere

"I read birth stories. It helped with my confidence. My fear was that I would 'wimp out.' But the more stories I read, the more confident I felt." – Amy

"I was scared in a way because I endured a lot of critical and unsupportive comments regarding my decision. Ultimately I learned not to talk about it with anyone, but I resolved to stay focused on the type of birth I wanted to have." – Bonnie

"[Most helpful during pregnancy was] reading positive birth stories and affirmations, instead of hearing about how painful it was." – April

"Ignore the negative stories everyone seems to want to tell you. Realize you were built to birth a baby without medical interventions." – Melanie

"[Most helpful during labor was] my mind set. I knew I didn't want pain meds so I never even gave it a thought. It just wasn't an option. I was just laboring like women have been doing for centuries." – Adriana

"[Most helpful during pregnancy was] tons of reading. Exposing myself to as many birth stories as possible (of all varieties!), mentally preparing myself...getting EXCITED

about birth! I think that makes the biggest difference; I don't fear the experience because I've learned to love it." – Bryn

When You Feel Capable, You Feel Courageous

It is important to recognize your innate capability to birth a baby naturally. Nourish that belief and your courage will grow.

** Discover any fears or concerns you may have; talk through them with your supportive caregiver, your partner, or trusted friends.

** Create a positive mental attitude using a variety of methods such as meditation, yoga, and/or affirmations.

** Maintain a positive atmosphere around you: only positive birth stories and people allowed!

My hope for you:

When labor starts you can face the upcoming hard work not with dread, doubt, and fear, but instead with confidence, excitement, and a sense of great purpose, saying to your baby: "It's my honor and privilege to bring you into the world."

"A woman in harmony with her spirit is like a river flowing. She goes where she will without pretense and arrives at her destination prepared to be herself and only herself." – Maya Angelou

I CAN AND I WILL

CHAPTER 5
PLAN AND PREPARE: A GREAT PARADOX OF BIRTH

"As for the future, your task is not to foresee it but to enable it." – Antoine de Saint Exupery

Planning and preparing, both mentally and physically, are very important to attaining a natural birth. A reminder about nature: it's not 100% guaranteed or predictable. Create your plans with your ideal birth vision in mind, provide all the right conditions for the birth to go perfectly, and then let go.

Your planning will set as many conditions in your favor as is possible and that you have control over. This planning and preparation will include the following:

    ** Attend a natural childbirth class.

    ** Create a birth plan.

    ** Prepare your body (and baby) for a natural birth.

Attend a Natural Childbirth Class

A very important part of preparing for a natural childbirth is to take a natural childbirth class. I recommend you attend the natural childbirth class with your partner, as he or she will play an important role in supporting you.

Knowledge helps dispel fear.

Regardless of the type of birth one wishes to have, it's very important to educate yourself about the birth process. However, a good natural childbirth class is more than just a collection of facts. It will:

** Provide education about the natural birth process.

** Build your confidence in your body's ability to give birth.

** Provide a place to discuss your concerns about labor and birth with an instructor as well as other couples in the class.

** Provide support and encouragement.

** Provide relaxation training as well as teach comfort and coping techniques.

** Provide a way for your partner to learn and be involved in the process.

** Provide information about interventions, when they are needed, and how to avoid them if they are not needed.

Word of Caution About Hospital-Based Birth Classes

When I talk about "natural childbirth classes" that's exactly what I mean – classes that teach preparation for an unmedicated childbirth. Do not confuse natural childbirth classes with simple "birth preparation" classes that are common at most hospitals.

These hospital-based classes aim to familiarize the parents-to-be with hospital policies and procedures and are intended to provide preparation for a typical hospital birth, which for most women includes getting pain relief in the form of an epidural. They will not help you prepare for your natural birth.

If you are birthing in a hospital and take the hospital-based birth class, I recommend also taking a natural childbirth class elsewhere.

Different Types Natural Childbirth Classes

There are many different natural childbirth classes available. Some offer a group setting with an instructor; others are self-study classes.

** The Bradley Method®

** Hypnobabies®

** HypnoBirthing®

** Lamaze®

** Birthing From Within®

** Hipbirth®

** Birth Works®

** Birth Boot Camp®

** Independent Classes

** The Pink Kit Method®

The Bradley Method® Natural Childbirth Classes

The Bradley Method (bradleybirth.com) is a comprehensive course that not only teaches methods of coping with labor pain, but also provides information about nutrition, staying healthy and low-risk, and relaxation exercises. This class also focuses on providing coaching training for your partner.

Bradley classes are held in small groups and taught by a trained Bradley instructor. There are usually 3-6 couples in a class, which usually meets once a week for 12 weeks.

According to their website, of the 1,000,000+ couples trained in The Bradley Method® nationwide, over 86% of them have had spontaneous, unmedicated vaginal births.

It is suggested to start taking Bradley classes in the fifth month.

To find a local Bradley instructor, you can ask your midwife or doctor, ask friends, conduct an online search in your area, or visit their website. (bradleybirth.com/Directory.aspx)

Sharing Stories: The Bradley Method

"[Most helpful about the class was that they were] evidence-based classes that taught active coping skills. I am a mover and I needed to have tools that worked with my need to be active." – Stacy

"[Most helpful about the class was] the positive nature of making natural birth seem attainable for average people." – Delilah

"There was such a wealth of information from signs of labor to delivery and recovery that my peers didn't receive from the 'traditional' pregnancy/birthing education." – D'Lynn

"They helped me understand how my body works. It gave me more control. I could know the pain was not abnormal. This decreased my fear. I also liked the fact that they involved the husbands so much. I didn't feel like I needed a doula because they prepared him so well." – Erin

"I also learned a lot about myself and how I deal with stress. I was able to develop a plan to use during labor to decrease my stress and that helped reduce pain." – Amy

Hypnobabies® Childbirth Hypnosis

Hypnobabies (hypnobabies.com) is a complete natural childbirth education course which teaches medical self-hypnosis techniques, adapted from master hypnotist Gerald Kein's Painless Childbirth Program, for a calm, relaxed, and comfortable labor and birth. These techniques allow the birthing mother to talk and move around during labor, and yet remain deeply in hypnosis.

As a comprehensive course, it also provides information about the physiology of birth, detailed birthing choices, optimal fetal positioning, nutrition, and staying healthy. (hypnobabies.com/classes/class-benefits)

Hypnobabies group classes are held for six weeks, three hours per week, and are taught by certified Hypnobabies instructors. To find a class near you, search their website. If there is not an instructor in your area, there is also a self-study course available.

The home-study course is a five-week course; expect to dedicate about 30-40 minutes each day for the course, plus an additional 35 minutes to listen to the daily affirmations. It's recommended to have at least two months or more to complete the course and practice the cues and techniques; starting around week 30 of your pregnancy is a good idea.

Visit their website for more information, to purchase the home study bundle (or additional audio tracks), or to locate a Hypnobabies instructor near you.

Sharing My Story

I took the Hypnobabies self-study course during my first pregnancy. It taught me how to remain calm, relaxed, and focused, which allowed my body to do what it needed to do. No tension, no fear. Because of that, labor progressed faster than normal for a first-time mom.

I loved the pregnancy affirmations. I believe they were key to really instilling a firm belief in myself and my body's ability to birth my baby naturally. The scripts that I practiced with my husband did a good job preparing him for supporting me.

Sharing Stories: Hypnobabies

"Hypnobabies helped to remind me pregnancy and birth are natural and our bodies were designed to do this." – *Melanie*

"Hypnobabies was excellent at providing me with everything I needed to know about childbirth and giving me tools that kept me completely comfortable and happy throughout the birth." – *Susan*

"Hypnobabies provided the structure I was looking for so I did that as a follow up [to HypnoBirthing]. I loved the audio track program." – *Anonymous*

"[Most helpful during pregnancy was my] daily practice of Hypnobabies cues." – *Dana*

HypnoBirthing® – The Mongan Method

HypnoBirthing (hypnobirthing.com) is another hypnosis-for-childbirth class. It is a philosophy of birth which teaches that in the absence of fear and tension, or special medical circumstances, severe pain does not have to be an accompaniment of labor—as taught by Dr. Grantly Dick-Read in the 1920s.

Classes teach you how to achieve the kind of relaxation (free of the resistance that fear creates) that allows the birthing muscles to work in harmony.

Classes are offered mainly through a HypnoBirthing practitioner. However, if there is not a practitioner in your area, there is learning material available on their website (book, CDs, and DVDs).

The class is taught in a series of five 2 ½-hour classes. To find a local

HypnoBirthing class, check their website. (hypnobirthing.com/directory)

Sharing Stories: HypnoBirthing

"[Most helpful about the class was] learning to connect into my husband's voice and the information about everything that goes on with birth." – Katie

"I left HypnoBirthing feeling a little unmoored, like I wasn't really sure what I was supposed to 'do.'" – Anonymous

Lamaze® International

Lamaze International (lamaze.org) is a nonprofit organization that promotes a natural, healthy, and safe approach to pregnancy, childbirth, and early parenting. The Lamaze Healthy Birth Practices are the foundation of Lamaze and include: spontaneous labor, walking and moving, continuous labor support, avoiding routine interventions, upright and spontaneous pushing, and keeping mother and baby together.

Lamaze classes focus on empowering women to trust in their body's natural design for birth and how to work with the body's natural abilities. They provide strategies for natural pain management during labor, which includes simple coping strategies, and breathing and movement techniques.

Lamaze classes are taught in groups of no more than 12 couples. To find a local Lamaze class, check their website. (lamaze.org/findalamazechildbirthclass) If there is no class near you, you can participate in an online class. (elearn.lamaze.org)

Birthing From Within®

A key feature of the Birthing From Within (birthingfromwithin.com) philosophy is the view that childbirth is a rite of passage. Viewing the purpose of childbirth preparation as awareness during birth, rather than achieving a specific birth outcome, there is acknowledgement that sometimes unexpected, unwelcome events may happen during labor.

Birthing From Within focuses on teaching expectant mothers and fathers to trust a woman's body. Classes include discussion about birth assumptions, emotional and physical preparation, pain coping techniques, and the role of the father in birth and breastfeeding. Classes include factual information, storytelling, and birth art.

Birthing From Within classes are taught in groups from a certified Birthing From Within mentor and usually meet once a week for six weeks. To find a local Birthing From Within class, check their website. (teachers.birthingfromwithin.com/teachers)

If there is no class near you, home study kits are available for purchase, as are private classes via phone or via Skype with either Pam England, the author of the book, or with Virginia Bobro, the programs director.

Hipbirth® The Childbirth Method

The Hipbirth Childbirth Method (hipbirth.com) focuses on relaxation, which helps remove stress hormones responsible for pain in childbirth as well as elevate endorphins. While promoting deep relaxation, the program also promotes movement.

The Hipbirth method is self-described as being a supplement to any childbirth preparation course you may be taking. According to their website, 80% of their clients give birth in less than six hours.

The program is structured as an online self-study course featuring video tutorials, guidebooks, and audio downloads. It is recommended to begin the program near your seventh month of pregnancy.

For more information or to purchase the program, visit their website. (hipbirth.com)

BirthWorks® International

BirthWorks (birthworks.org) believes that birth is instinctive and that women don't need to be taught how to birth but rather how to have more faith and trust in their own ability to give birth. The aim is to decrease fear and increase confidence.

BirthWorks classes provide physical and emotional preparation for birth including exploring human values, providing opportunities for grieving and healing, pelvic bodywork, labor comfort measures, nutrition and exercise, optimal fetal positioning, breastfeeding, and postpartum care. The entire class outline is on their website.

It is recommended to take BirthWorks class early in pregnancy, or even before pregnancy, since that is a good time for exploring beliefs about birth.

To find a local BirthWorks class, check their website. (birthworks.org/find-a-child-birth-class)

Birth Boot Camp®

Birth Boot Camp (birthbootcamp.com) is a complete natural childbirth education course that not only teaches methods of coping with labor pain and relaxation exercises, but also provides information about nutrition; staying healthy, strong, and low-risk; physiology of birth; birthing choices; and birth locations and support. This class also provides training for your partner. There is also an extra class on breastfeeding.

Birth Boot Camp group classes are held once a week for 10 weeks and are taught by certified Birth Boot Camp instructors. To find a class near you, search their website. If there is not an instructor in your area, there is also an online course available. (birthbootcamp.com/find-a-live-childbirth-class)

It is recommended to start Birth Boot Camp classes as close to 28 weeks as possible.

Independent Natural Childbirth Classes

Some doulas or other trained childbirth educators offer their own natural childbirth classes. They may incorporate a variety of different coping techniques (e.g., Bradley, Lamaze, Birthing From Within, HypnoBirthing, etc.) instead of focusing on a single method. They may take place weekly for several weeks or may be held in a one weekend "boot camp" style.

As an independent instructor, one who is not associated with a certain care provider or institution, they are able to provide candid answers that other instructors may not be able to do. Some may even offer faith-based classes. Keep in mind, though, that independent childbirth educators may or may not be actually certified with each type of natural childbirth method they discuss.

To find an independent natural childbirth class, try an online search for classes in your area.

Sharing Stories: Independent Classes

"[The instructor] tailored it to the type of births each of the members in the class wanted to have. Those seeking natural births would really be helped by knowing what to look for with pain. And those in a hospital setting who wanted to go natural would be well-served to know about all the interventions and their options and how it usually goes in a hospital." – Delayna

"[Most helpful about the class was learning] how to talk/deal with hospital doctors and staff about having a 'low-intervention' birth. – Jen

The Pink Kit Method®

The Pink Kit Method (thepinkkit.com) is a skills-based childbirth preparation that helps you prepare your body for birth. The information provided will help you discover and map your own specific pelvic anatomy, which will help you prepare for the route your baby will take on the way out. Also included is information about body positioning and several techniques for creating space. You can purchase the kit on their website. (thepinkkit.com/the-pink-kit-package-digital-download)

Sharing Stories: General Thoughts on Group Classes

"[I didn't like] 'labor rehearsal' in front of people where we were supposed to lay down on the floor and go through guided relaxation with our husband massaging us. It was awkward and embarrassing." – Delilah

"I appreciated the discussions, questions, and concerns that were brought up by the couples. … Listening to real people share and ask questions creates a sense of community that made the childbirth class a wonderful experience." – Samantha

"I met other people with the same philosophy. I was able to think, 'I'm not different than her. If she can do it, I can do it.' It was a great support group." – Amy

Create a Birth Plan: Your Ideal Birth Vision

A birth plan is a written list of your preferences for different aspects of your labor, birth, and newborn care. It is intended as a means of communicating your birthing preferences to your caregiver and the staff who will be attending your birth, especially when your preferences differ from the common practices they may use.

Keep in mind that birth is of nature and therefore cannot be completely planned. You can set the stage, provide all the right conditions (that are in your control), but then you must step back, let go, and let nature happen.

With that in mind, you may want to think of your birth plan as your **ideal birth vision**.

Why Create a Birth Plan?

"Reduce your plan to writing. The moment you complete this, you will have definitely given concrete form to the intangible desire." – Napoleon Hill

Reasons to create a birth plan include:

** Provide an **exercise in researching all your birthing options**, many of which you may not even be aware of, and putting your preferences into writing. The information you gather will help you think about what you want your birth to be like, as well as highlight some things that you may not want. As the saying goes, if you don't know your choices then you don't have any.

** Provide an **avenue to discuss birthing options with your caregiver** during pregnancy. You will learn if your caregiver is supportive of your preferences and may find out if any of your preferences cannot or will not be honored during birth. If your caregiver is not completely supportive of your plan, especially in an area that really matters to you, it's better to find this information out now when you have time to find a new provider or birthing location.

Birth plans are not mandates. There is no guarantee that your doctor, hospital, or care provider will follow your plan, even if they initially seem accepting of it.

What Goes in a Birth Plan?

A birth plan can include your preferences (what you want, don't want, or will refuse) on the following topics:

   ** Monitoring of labor (continuous EFM or intermittent fetal monitoring)

   ** Hydration/nutrition (eat or drink as desired)

   ** Pain management preferences

   ** Environment (music, privacy/minimal interruptions, dim lighting)

   ** Comfort items (own clothing, own pillow, people present)

   ** Medical procedure preferences (IV fluids, induction, augmentation, episiotomy, instrument delivery)

   ** Freedom of movement (use the birth ball, use tub or shower,

walking, rocking)
** Pushing positions (freedom to choose position when ready)
** Unexpected events (including medical interventions or cesarean)
** Postpartum and newborn care (Pitocin, cord clamping, breastfeeding, rooming in or nursery, circumcision or intact, eye drops, vitamin K)
** Desire for informed consent (risks, benefits, consequences of refusal, and alternatives are to be discussed before every procedure on yourself and your baby)

When to Create a Birth Plan

You can create a birth plan whenever you decide on your birth preferences, keeping in mind that your preferences may change throughout your pregnancy.

Aiming to complete your birth plan around the sixth month of pregnancy (around week 26) is a good idea. That should give you enough time to do some research, but also be enough time to discuss your birth plan with your provider. If your care provider does not support certain aspects of your plan, you may need time to consider your options.

How to Write a Birth Plan

I recommend writing two birth plans:
** One **detailed plan** that lists all your preferences on all the topics mentioned previously. This is your ideal birth vision, everything you want and care about, on one page. This detailed plan is for **you and your partner**, as well as for discussion with your care provider during pregnancy. You can bring this to the birth location for your own reference, but I recommend against giving hospital staff this one.
** One **simple plan**, perhaps just a few sentences, to **bring to your birthing site** when you are in labor. This is your respectful request for their support of your natural birth.

There are many websites that provide information about writing detailed birth plans; here is one to start (and one for fun):
** **BirthingNaturally:** Provides birth plan options (birthingnaturally.net/birthplan/options/options.html), checklist (great list of options that may help you start your research) (birthingnaturally.net/forms/birthplan.pdf), sample birth plans, and formats (birthingnaturally.net/birthplan/sample/index.html).
** **Midwiferytoday:** I enjoyed the humor in this one. (midwiferytoday.com/articles/birthplan.asp)

Here are a few sample detailed birth plans, which may help you in forming your own:
** Sample One (s3.amazonaws.com/BlogPDFs/My-Natural-Birth-Preferences.pdf)
** Sample Two (thehumbledhomemaker.com/2012/08/a-sample-hospital-birth-plan.html)

** Sample Three, Bradley Method birth plan (lifeyourway.net/our-bradley-method-birth-plan)

** Sample Four (alternative-mama.com/how-to-write-a-birth-plan)

** Sample Five, excellent ideas for simple, bulleted, easy to read (ncbi.nlm.nih.gov/pmc/articles/PMC1948092/figure/fig2)

For a simple plan consider using one of the following sentences, perhaps together with a lovely photo or drawing and placed on the hospital room door:

** We appreciate your support in our goal of a natural birth.

** Please help me achieve the most natural birth possible.

** Natural birth in progress. Thank you for your support and encouragement!

Advice Regarding Birth Plans

No one likes to be told what to do, especially before they've been given a chance to support you. If you decide to create a birth plan for the hospital staff, keep it simple (bulleted list), short (one page), and sweet (respectful language, phrased positively). You have more chance of the hospital staff reading (and hopefully honoring) your wishes if it's quick and easy for them to read.

Think of statements starting with, "Thank you for..." and "I would prefer...", instead of "Do not ever...".

For example:

** Write: "I would like labor to begin naturally," instead of "No Pitocin."

** Write: "Please use a hand-held Doppler or fetoscope to monitor baby's heart rate," instead of "No continuous EFM."

** Write: "Thank you for using soft voices and keeping the lights low," instead of "No loud talking or bright lights."

** Write: "Encouragement and support is welcome, especially if I look like I am in pain," instead of "Do not offer pain medication."

I recommend giving people the benefit of the doubt, expecting that they will respect your wish for a natural birth and be happy to support you in that goal. Give them a chance to support you, you may be pleasantly surprised.

Sharing Stories: Birth Plans for Hospitals

My friend Juliana birthed all four of her children naturally in a hospital and she chose not to have a formal written birth plan. Instead, what she found very helpful was putting a sign on the outside of her hospital room door which pictured two women wrapped in robes and contained the text, "Natural birth in progress. Do not offer drugs or interventions."

"If you are going the hospital/OB route, write a BRIEF birth plan and discuss it with your OB. Be aware you are asking hospital staff to do something that may be well

outside their comfort zone. BE NICE TO THEM." – Kate

Birth Plan for a Natural Birth at Home or a Birth Center

It's always a good exercise to create a birth plan for the reasons mentioned previously.

If you are birthing at home or at a birth center with a midwife, she may be more inclined to naturally have similar views as you do on birth; however, not all midwives have the same birth philosophy. You will discover her birth philosophy and practices as you progress through your pregnancy, and especially when you discuss your birth plan. This is when you can discuss and note any of your preferences that deviate from her standard birth practices.

Sharing My Story: Birth Plan for Birth Center and Home Birth

I chose to see a midwife at a birth center. During my first pregnancy I started to create a birth plan but, during discussions with my midwife throughout pregnancy, I realized what I was putting in the plan was part of her birth philosophy as well as the normal birth practices of the birth center: our views on labor, birth, and postpartum care were completely synced. I ended up not writing a birth plan for either of my births, and instead just noted the few newborn procedures I was refusing.

Preparing Your Body (and Baby) for a Natural Birth

While you can't control everything during pregnancy and birth, there are a few things you can do that may help set the stage for a natural birth:
    ** Practice excellent nutrition.
    ** Get enough and appropriate exercise.
    ** Learn and implement optimal baby positioning.
    ** Get regular chiropractic adjustments.
    ** Prepare the birth canal.
    ** Uterus toning and cervical ripening.

Practice Excellent Nutrition

"No amount of prenatal blood sampling, uterine testing, ultrasounds, amniocentesis, or other physical evaluations can substitute for good maternal nutrition." – Dr. David Stewart

Contrary to widespread myth, pregnancy is not the time to abandon healthy eating and devour junk food in the name of "more calories." In order to avoid health-related complications that could affect your health, your baby's health, and your natural birth, it is wise to practice excellent prenatal nutrition.

Hopefully your caregiver is providing nutritional education and counseling at your prenatal appointments, as this has been shown to have health benefits for the mother as well as the baby.

Benefits of excellent prenatal nutrition:

 ** Have a healthy weight baby.

 ** Prevent pre-term birth.

 ** Prevent preeclampsia.

 ** Grow a strong and healthy placenta.

 ** Achieve adequate iron levels.

 ** Maintain flexible and elastic perineum.

 ** Postpartum recovery (makes it faster and easier).

What is excellent prenatal nutrition? I will leave the details for you to research and discuss with your caregiver, but the basics include eating high-quality foods from all the food groups, with enough protein, healthy fats, adequate salt (to taste), and filtered water (to thirst), while reducing empty-calorie junk foods. Think real foods, as close to their original state as possible (not processed), lots of colors, lots of variety.

Here are two sources for healthy pregnancy diets that you may want to read and then discuss with your caregiver:

 ** **The Brewer Diet:** Dr. Tom Brewer created guidelines for prenatal nutrition that he credits for helping his patients achieve optimal health (preventing preeclampsia and Toxemia). therealblueribbonbaby.org

 ** **Weston A. Price Foundation:** This diet for pregnant and nursing mothers has some similar components to the Brewer Diet, with a few added ones as well as a list of what to avoid. westonaprice.org/health-topics/diet-for-pregnant-and-nursing-mothers

Sharing My Story

After reviewing my food journal in early pregnancy, my midwife and I discussed many aspects of a healthy diet, including appropriate protein intake during pregnancy and healthy foods that would help maintain my iron levels.

I took a few supplements such as a whole food-based prenatal vitamin, cod liver oil, digestive enzymes, probiotics, and others as needed.

In addition to eating many healthy vegetables, enough protein, healthy fats (avocado, olive oil, coconut oil, nuts, seeds), and lots of filtered water, I went beyond typical recommendations in the name of achieving optimal health during this special growing time. I eliminated all processed sugar and caffeine, reduced empty-calorie junk carbohydrates, and drank a healthy greens powder mixed with water.

I also kept following the many other healthy eating and lifestyle choices that we had previously incorporated into our lives and that I believe are important. You may want to research these areas yourself if you are interested, but here are other things I did for optimal health:

 ** Eliminated tuna

** Drank a glass of lemon water first thing in the morning

** Avoided artificial sweeteners, high fructose corn syrup, MSG, artificial food colorings, and other food additives and preservatives

** Cooked only with stainless steel or glass (no Teflon)

** Stored food in glass containers only (no plastic)

** Did not use microwave to heat food (heated on stove top or in oven)

** Drank only filtered water (no fluoride or other chemicals)

** Drank out of glass or stainless steel containers

** Ate only organic food

** Used personal care products with better ingredients (soap, shampoo, toothpaste, deodorant)

My iron levels stayed quite healthy the entire pregnancy, my amniotic sac did not rupture until very active labor (around 9-10cm dilation), my babies had a very healthy birth weight, I had no problems with bleeding after the birth, I felt great immediately after birth, and I recovered quickly. I credit a lot of that to my healthy diet as well as staying active.

Get Enough and Appropriate Exercise

Women who exercise during pregnancy handle the work of labor easier, tend to have shorter labors, have an easier time pushing baby out, need fewer medical interventions, and physically recover easier.

Exercise can prepare the pelvic floor muscles for birth, as can Kegel exercises (pelvic floor contractions). Doing Kegel exercises during pregnancy has been associated with easier labors.

Talk to your health care provider before starting any exercise program during pregnancy. You may need to modify your current exercise plan as your pregnancy progresses; your care provider can help you determine when modifications are necessary as well as provide alternatives.

Generally, walking and prenatal yoga are considered safe. Running and swimming provide good exercise if you are cleared for such activities.

Sharing My Story

I am a runner and I continued to run during my pregnancies; until 30 weeks with my first pregnancy and until 26 weeks with my second pregnancy. I also lifted weights. When I stopped running, I used the elliptical machine and went for daily walks.

If you run (and even if you walk) I recommend using a maternity support band/belt. It helps support a growing belly and removes some of the pressure that a growing belly can place on the pelvic joints.

Sharing Stories: Staying Healthy

"Going to the hospital was my biggest fear and by making my health a priority

throughout pregnancy, I managed to avoid any issues that would have required interventions." – Angela

"I remained active throughout all three of my pregnancies. I continued to work out on a regular basis up to my deliveries and feel that it gave me the stamina to give birth and allowed for smooth/quick deliveries with fast recovery time." – Tatiana

"[Most helpful during pregnancy was] reading literature, yoga, meditation, and continuing to be active throughout the pregnancy. I felt strong the entire pregnancy." – Andrea

"Staying physically active was most helpful." – Grace

Learn and Implement Optimal Baby Positioning

The position of the baby's head and body can affect how the cervix opens and the ease of the baby's rotation and descent. If the baby is in a good position when labor starts, there is a higher chance of a smooth delivery.

The optimal fetal position for spontaneous vaginal delivery is Left Occiput Anterior (LOA), which means the baby is head down with its back on the mom's left side and the back of the baby's head (occiput) is facing the mother's front (anterior). A baby with the back of their head towards mom's back (posterior) or head up (breech) may present a challenge.

When your caregiver starts palpating your abdomen to determine baby's position, ask what position baby is in and note it. Baby's position can and will change throughout the pregnancy, so there is no need to panic if baby is not in optimal position at 26 weeks.

A baby can find an optimal position earlier in pregnancy (once it turns head down) or it can wait until the end of pregnancy or even labor to find that position. For example, most posterior babies rotate in labor.

Trust your baby. The baby will naturally know how to find the easiest path out.

You Can Help Baby's Position

While it's no guarantee, certain prenatal postures, positions, and exercises can help your baby find an optimal position for an easier birth. There are also certain maternal postures and positions that can hinder your baby's position.

** Watch your posture when sitting. When you sit in a chair sit on the edge with your knees below your hips, or sit on a firm exercise ball that allows your hips to be higher than your knees.

** Watch your posture when resting. No reclining backward (especially with your feet elevated) or lying on your back after 20 weeks. Your baby's head and spine are the heaviest part of their body and will flow and rotate with gravity. When you recline your baby will rotate so the heaviest part of their body will be down.

** Sleep on your left side. Baby's head/spine should roll into a nice

LOA position.

** Get regular chiropractic adjustments. If certain ligaments are too tight, it restricts the baby's movements in the uterus and they may not be able to get into a good position. Monthly adjustments are highly recommended, and they can increase to every 2-3 weeks towards the end of pregnancy.

Visit the Spinning Babies website for more information about baby position, maternal positions, and techniques to help baby move to an optimal position. (spinningbabies.com)

Sharing My Story

I practiced proper baby positioning posture, as mentioned above, with both pregnancies.

With my first pregnancy, my son always presented LOA and once he was in that position, he never changed. Labor followed a regular pattern and his birth was smooth; I was able to breathe him out.

With my second pregnancy my daughter always presented posterior, usually Right Occiput Posterior (ROP). Labor with my daughter started slower, stopping and starting over a long day, possibly due to her posterior position.

After my daughter was born my midwife said she started presenting posterior, but when her head was showing quite a bit, she turned 180 degrees and ended up being born anterior. And from my point of view, I couldn't feel anything different. My baby figured the smoothest way out.

Sharing a Story

My friend Juliana birthed her first three babies posteriorly (and naturally at a hospital). Her doctor then told her that there was no way she would ever have a baby present in the optimal (anterior) position due to her pelvis shape. During her pregnancy with her fourth baby she learned about posture and its effect on baby's position. Reflecting on her favorite relaxation positions during her first three pregnancies, she realized she always sat back with her knees pulled to her chest, or reclined back with her feet propped up. Determined to do what she could do this time around she focused on keeping her belly down and forward while sitting, keeping her knees below her hips, and she did not recline backwards. When she went into labor with her fourth baby, the baby presented anteriorly and was born easily and smoothly as Juliana breathed her out.

Changing a Breech Presentation

Most care providers will recommend a cesarean if the baby is presenting in a breech position towards the end of pregnancy or at the start of labor. Since your goal is a natural childbirth, you will want to learn your options if your baby is in a breech position towards the end of pregnancy.

Keep in mind that breech babies can and have turned on their own even as late as 36 weeks and beyond. So if it's much earlier in your pregnancy, there's no need to panic.

There are several different options that have been effective in turning a breech baby toward the end of pregnancy:

** The Spinning Babies website has some ideas for turning a breech baby. Some of the most common methods include pelvic tilts, hip openers, inclines, forward leaning inversions, Rebozo sifting, visualization, and talking to your baby. (spinningbabies.com)

** Moxibustion has been also used successfully to turn breech babies, especially if used around week 34. A form of Traditional Chinese Medicine, moxibustion is an externally applied treatment using the dry leaves of the mugwort plant compressed and rolled into cigar-shaped sticks. These Moxa sticks are lit and held near an acupuncture point near the edge of the outer toe. The heat from the burning Moxa sticks can stimulate baby's movement and encourage it to turn.

** The chiropractic Webster Technique has also been used successfully to turn breech babies. It is a specific adjustment used to help balance the mother's pelvis, relieving tense muscles and ligaments which may be preventing the baby from being in an optimal position. It is performed by chiropractors certified in the technique.

** External Cephalic Version (ECV) is a procedure that externally rotates a breech baby to a vertex (head down) position. The procedure is performed by a doctor at or after 37 weeks (full term) because there is a chance the procedure can start labor. If labor starts and baby is breech, a cesarean can be performed. Since it is quite an involved procedure it is often used as a last resort if others methods to turn baby have not worked.

Get Regular Chiropractic Adjustments

Routine chiropractic care can be helpful for comfort during pregnancy, but it can also reduce labor time. When a baby presents in the optimal (anterior) position, labor and birth can proceed smoothly.

Chiropractic adjustments can keep the pelvis in balance, which keeps the ligaments connected to the uterus in balance. A misaligned pelvis can reduce the amount of room available for the developing baby as well as make it harder for baby to get into the best position for delivery.

There is a specific chiropractic adjustment for pregnant women, called the Webster Technique, in which the chiropractor can establish balance in the pelvis and connecting ligaments. This balanced state promotes optimal fetal positioning which in turn leads to a safer, easier birth.

The International Chiropractic Pediatric Association (ICPA) provides a website that has more information on this topic. To find a chiropractor certified in the Webster Technique and who specializes in prenatal care, pregnancy, and children, use the locator on their website. (icpa4kids.org/Find-a-Chiropractor)

Sharing My Story

I got regular chiropractic adjustments throughout both my pregnancies. I went monthly until the last few months when I started going every 2-3 weeks. It kept me comfortable; I didn't have any of the common pregnancy aches and pains. I also believe it helped my births go smoothly.

Sharing a Story

"[Most important during pregnancy was] chiropractic care and visits with [my] midwife." – Rosa

Prepare the Birth Canal, Protect the Perineum

If you are nervous about pushing baby out, or possibly tearing your perineum (the delicate area between the vagina and anus) in doing so, I want to share a few tips that might enable a smoother delivery and recovery. Whether these actions directly help or not it can feel empowering to know you did everything you could do to prepare. You may then be more able to let go and approach the birth with more confidence.

** **Perineal massage:** Some studies have shown that performing a perineal massage in the last few weeks of pregnancy can help prevent tearing during birth, especially for first-time moms. A perineal massage is performed daily by you in the privacy of your own home. It involves inserting two lubricated fingers and stretching the lower vaginal wall.

** **Exercise:** Some say perineal massage is old-fashioned and not necessary, and that regular exercise is effective in preparing and strengthening the perineal area.

** **Kegels:** Kegels are pelvic floor contractions that help make your pelvic floor stronger and more elastic, which can help during birth.

** **Nutrition:** As mentioned previously, excellent prenatal nutrition can help with skin elasticity. For details, check out this article from BirthFaith.org on protecting the perineum from the inside out. (http://birthfaith.org/nutrition/protecting-your-perineum-from-the-inside-out)

** **Birth Position:** The side-lying (lateral) position has been shown to be the birth position with the highest rate of intact perineum.

Sharing My Story

I had an intact perineum with both of my births (did not tear). I exercised throughout both pregnancies (running, elliptical machine, walking) and did Kegels. I did perineal massage during the last few weeks of my first pregnancy but not at all during my second. For both of my births I pushed in a lateral position.

Uterus Toning and Cervical Ripening

There are several traditional herbal supplements that are favorites in the midwifery world for toning the uterus and preparing the cervix for a smoother labor: red raspberry leaf tea and evening primrose oil. However, there are very few studies on consuming them during pregnancy. They appear to be safe for mother and baby, but you should always consult your care provider before taking this or any other supplement while pregnant.

    ** **Red raspberry leaf tea:** Drinking red raspberry leaf tea in late pregnancy is believed to tone the uterus and help make the contractions more effective during labor. As an astringent herb, it may help prevent excessive bleeding after childbirth.

    ** **Evening primrose oil:** Evening Primrose Oil (EPO) contains gamma-linoleic acids which the body converts to prostaglandins. Taking EPO capsules late in pregnancy is believed to help ripen the cervix, due to the actions of the prostaglandins produced.

    ** **Dates:** Eating dates during the last month of pregnancy may help shorten labor as well as reduce the need for induction or augmentation of labor. Study participants who ate six dates a day for the last four weeks of pregnancy had higher cervical dilation upon admission and had labors that were approximately 6.5 hours shorter than the non-date eating participants. (They also had a higher proportion of intact membranes and spontaneous labor.)

Sharing My Story

Starting at 36 or 37 weeks, I started drinking several cups of red raspberry leaf tea daily, which is caffeine free. Also at 36 or 37 weeks, I started inserting 1000mg of EPO capsules vaginally before bed. (Tip: Body heat will melt the capsules, so wearing a panty liner is recommended.)

    While I cannot say that the red raspberry leaf tea or EPO directly affected my labor or birth, I can say that I had very straightforward labors and births. I went into labor right around 40 weeks exactly both times. I had no trouble dilating or effacing and no problems with bleeding after the birth.

The Paradox of Natural Birth: Plan and Prepare

A great paradox of natural birth is that by relinquishing control to the forces of nature—by letting go and letting the waves come and do their job —you can end up with a birth where you feel mastery and that you were actually the one in control. But that doesn't mean you should sit back and do nothing to prepare.

    While you can't control all of what happens during labor and birth, you can make choices that set the stage for your ideal birth.

** Attending a natural childbirth class will help you gain information and confidence in a supportive environment.

** Creating a birth plan will help you learn your childbirth options and provide a means of discussing them with your care provider.

** Preparing your body by eating well, exercising, and maintaining good posture can help enable a smooth labor and birth.

"Confidence is preparation. Everything else is beyond your control." – Richard Kline

I CAN AND I WILL

PART 2: COMFORT STRATEGIES DURING LABOR

"There is the mud, and there is the lotus that grows out of the mud. We need the mud in order to make the lotus." – Thich Nhat Hanh

There are some ideas floating around that promise a pain-free or very fast labor. And while that can indeed happen, I believe the percentage of women who feel no pain or have extremely short labors is very small, especially for first-time moms.

It is important to have realistic expectations about labor and birth. You may wonder what that means if you've never given birth before. Simply put, expect the following:

    ** There will be pain.

    ** It will probably last for a while.

    ** You can handle it.

    ** It will be worth it.

This section of the book contains wisdom that worked for me in coping with the pain, not eliminating the pain during labor.

In general, throughout labor you will want to find ways to maintain:

    ** autonomy

    ** privacy

    ** comfort

    ** support

Sharing Stories:

"I knew it would be painful but I had to prepare my mind and body for something that it was designed to do." – Amber

"Pain during labor is temporary. It can be managed with breathing techniques and great coaching." – Grace

"Keep an open mind as well and do your research so that you are better prepared and have various methods to use when things get intense." – Tatiana

"Realize there will be some pain but nothing you can't handle. And believe in yourself." – Monique

CHAPTER 6
LABOR AT HOME AS LONG AS POSSIBLE

"Be patient. You'll know when it's time for you to wake up and move ahead." –
Ram Dass

Despite what you may have seen on TV or in the movies, most labors do not start with your water breaking (only about 8% do) nor is there quite the need to rush to the hospital, as labors can last an average of 16 hours for first-time moms.

Labors can start in many different ways and progress in many different ways. The factors involved can range from number of births you've previously had (if any) to the position of the baby to genetic factors to other variables.

Laboring at home as long as possible is beneficial for ensuring a natural childbirth. Unless it is medically indicated otherwise, plan to labor at home at home as long as possible.

Why Does Laboring at Home Help Natural Childbirth?

At home you are free to labor as you like, depending on how you feel. You are surrounded by comfort and a familiar environment: your bed, your sofa, your shower, your pajamas, your pictures on the wall, your family. When you are relaxed and in a calm, comfortable, and safe environment, your body can relax and labor more efficiently.

Once admitted to the hospital, you are entering their territory with all their policies, which may or may not support natural birth, as discussed previously. The earlier in labor you arrive at the hospital the longer you have to be in this unfamiliar environment. Gone are your comforts of home, replaced with people you don't know, bright lights, many interruptions, and other such things that may interfere with creating a safe and comfortable environment.

You will also probably be "on the clock," meaning they will be expecting you to deliver your baby in a certain amount of time (or at a time convenient to them) and if they deem your labor too long, may impose actions that you may not want.

By waiting until later in labor, maybe 6-8 cm dilated, you will be arriving at the birth location with less time until birth. That is, less time to allow any uncomfortable surroundings to affect your labor. You have had time to find your labor rhythm, labor is in full swing, and you are almost done.

Activities for Early Labor

Depending on how your labor starts, your contractions may be far apart and not that strong at first and you may have many hours to spend at home laboring. You may want to plan ahead for what you can do during this time.

Here are a few good activities for early labor:
** Tend to regular daily tasks or make any last-minute preparations, depending on how you feel.
** Go for a walk. Gravity helps the baby's head push against the cervix to help it dilate.
** Take a shower; the warm water feels great.
** Watch a favorite show; it is a great way to relax and pass the time, especially if the show is a comedy.
** Listen to music. Whatever keeps your mind in a positive state is a good thing.
** Call a friend to chat. Talking to someone can help pass the time as well as take your mind off the contractions.
** Eat and drink as you feel. Nourish your body for the work ahead.

You may want to work on a special project during this time. Having a focused activity may help keep your mind occupied with something besides the contractions, with the added benefit of accomplishing a task!

Sharing My Story

I laugh about my planned activity for early labor with my first child! I was sure early contractions would be 20+ minutes apart so I planned to spend early labor working on the birth announcements. I purchased the needed materials ahead of time (scrapbook paper and coordinating ribbon) and planned to spend early labor cutting the paper and assembling it into the announcements. I thought it was a great plan, a great use of time, and a great way to distract myself.

Once labor started, all those plans went out the window very quickly.

While not very strong at first, the contractions were 5-10 minutes apart from the get-go and all I felt like doing was lying on the couch and listening to my Hypnobabies CDs. (The birth announcements didn't get assembled until our son was about six weeks old.)

You can have a plan for early labor, but be prepared to change your mind once labor starts. You never know how it's going to go or what you will feel like doing!

When to Head to the Birth Facility

Your care provider should discuss their protocol for when to call or when to head to the birth location, which would include their instructions for certain situations such as your water breaking or for emergencies.

In general aim to call your provider and head to the birth location once you are in active labor, which may present with these signs:

** Contractions are 3-5 minutes apart, lasting for one minute or longer, and have been so for one hour.

** You are not talking between contractions, or you need help to focus through each one.

Sharing Stories: Laboring at Home

"If you are going to a hospital spend a long period [laboring] at home. Once you are there, you'll [be] less comfortable. [Most helpful during labor was] staying home from the hospital as long as possible. Being in a safe comfortable zone." – Jenny

"[Most helpful during labor was] pretending like I wasn't in labor as long as possible. – Rachel

One Tip to Maintain Privacy

I know this may not be popular advice in our current society of share-everything-you-are-doing-the-instant-you-are-doing-it, but here goes:

Only let the people directly involved with your birth know that you are in labor.

Maybe it's the introvert in me, but we only notified one person that I was in labor with our first child (our midwife) and two people with our second child (our midwife and our birth photographer).

Unless they are needed to help with the care of older children or are involved in supporting you during the birth, I would wait and surprise family and friends with a phone call when your baby is born.

Why?

I didn't want anyone hanging on for more information, updates, or status reports. I didn't want certain people worrying about me. I didn't want to feel like I was on some sort of time clock. I didn't want people constantly calling to check in, taking my focus away (or my husband's).

I wanted that space to have our birth together. Just us. No outside pressure, real or imagined.

Let your labor be about you and your partner and your baby. The rest of the world can be notified when the time is right.

"However much we know about birth in general, we know nothing about a particular birth. We must let it unfold with its own uniqueness." – Elizabeth Noble

CHAPTER 7
TURN FEAR INTO ACCEPTANCE

"Vulnerability is our most accurate measure of courage." – Brené Brown

Fear affects labor.

Laboring without fear or anxiety is a very important key to having a natural birth.

Fear-Tension-Pain Cycle

The uterus has two opposing muscle layers that work together during labor. When we are afraid our body releases adrenaline, and during labor that can affect the function of the uterus muscles, causing them to work in opposition, with one muscle layer trying to open the cervix and the other muscle layer trying to close the cervix. This slows the progress of labor: each contraction is less effective, meaning less dilation. And that will result in a longer, harder labor, which will make your dream of natural birth harder to achieve.

Thus, fear during labor results in what Dr. Grantly Dick-Read termed the "Fear-Tension-Pain" cycle.

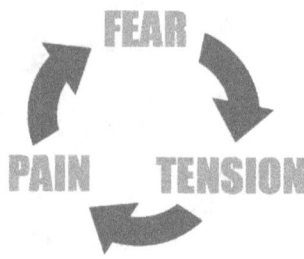

Fear of, or resistance to, what is happening will lead to tension in your body. Tension in your body will lead to increased pain. Increased pain leads to more fear, and so the cycle continues.

The birthing muscles work in perfect harmony when your body is relaxed. Labor is faster when you aren't fighting your body or what is happening.

Let the knowledge of the Fear-Tension-Pain cycle serve as a guide to do whatever it takes to help you feel safe, calm, and relaxed during labor.

    ** Choose or create a birthing environment that feels safe and protective.

    ** Learn to deeply relax physically, mentally, and emotionally.

Create a Calm and Safe Environment

As all mammals do, we need to feel safe and protected during birth. Those who work closely with animals know they prefer a birthing environment that is quiet, dark, safe, and familiar, with space to move as they wish.

If you are not birthing at home, here are a few things to consider in order to create a calm, safe, and private birthing area:

    ** Have dim lighting.

    ** Listen to quiet music.

    ** Make sure room has only pleasing smells.

    ** Bring your own pillow, blanket, or other comfort items.

    ** Wear your own clothing, whatever is comfortable.

Even though it seems harmless, putting on a hospital gown can have an effect on the laboring woman. Being forced to wear something you did not choose and are not comfortable in may lead you to feel as if you are giving your power to the hospital, or perhaps even losing some your confidence in your ability to birth on your own terms.

Sharing Stories: Calm Environment

"[Most helpful during labor was] laboring in the water, in a quiet, non-invasive environment." – April

"[Most helpful during labor was] being at home where I was relaxed and calm." – Amy

Check for Tension and Release It

Your partner may want to periodically check your tension levels.

    ** Do your arms, face, legs, or forehead tighten during a contraction?

    ** Is your mouth clenched?

    ** Are you shrieking or screaming in a high-pitched, shallow, almost panicked way?

Tension in other parts of your body means tension in your birthing muscles. You may be resisting the contraction and may need a reminder to "relax here."

Famous midwife Ina May Gaskin notes a connection between tension in the mouth and jaw and tension in the cervix. If you find your mouth or jaw pursed tight or clenched, chances are the same is happening with your cervix. Focus on relaxing your mouth (and your cervix) by making noise like a horse (flapping your lips while exhaling) or by kissing your partner.

Let It All Out

Releasing emotions is another good way to relieve tension. Laughing, crying, complaining, moaning, and swearing can be beneficial for a release. You may need to express your pain rather than act as if it doesn't hurt.

Being in a safe and comfortable environment will help you feel uninhibited, so you can express yourself as needed.

Sharing My Story

Knowing about the fear-tension-pain cycle helped me so much. If I noticed that I was tensing up during a contraction, I changed that fear to focus. I focused on relaxing and letting the contraction happen. I focused on my husband's gentle, softly spoken words during each contraction. Throughout each contraction, he would repeatedly say:

    ** release the energy

    ** peace

    ** relax

    ** breathe and release

During a contraction I focused on breathing out the energy; I exhaled deeply and purposefully. I found that keeping my breathing deep and low, with added moans and vocalization when necessary, helped to release the energy of the contraction.

By breathing through the contractions and letting them happen, I was able to be deeply relaxed. Which I believed help me have a fairly quick labor, especially for a first-time mom.

Sharing Stories: Staying Relaxed

"Read up on birth without fear, and understand that our bodies have a wonderful system of minimizing the pain of birth if we don't allow fear and tension to take over." – Elanna

"[Most helpful during labor was] horselips!!! (See Ina May)" – Alicia

"[Most helpful during labor was] having a supportive midwife, laboring at home, having my husband confident in me, and having confidence in myself so I could stay relaxed! Staying relaxed and trusting that my body would produce natural pain-coping hormones helped immensely." – Kristen

"[Most helpful during labor was] letting my body do what it needed to do without any interference." – Kimberly

Focus on Accepting What is Happening

"Rain, after all, is only rain; it is not bad weather. So also, pain is only pain; unless we resist it, then it becomes torment." – I Ching

You can get in the way of yourself and your progress by resisting each contraction; wanting to eliminate it, shorten it, or wish it wasn't so hard or long. Change your focus to accepting each contraction. When you **accept each contraction** and let your body do what it knows how to do, the **labor will be faster and smoother**.

Your goal through each contraction is to be so completely and deeply relaxed that your body can do what it needs to do most efficiently.

Acceptance means relinquishing control of your body to nature and being okay with what is. Be vulnerable and surrender completely to the process of birth.

But you are not without control, for you are always in control of your mind.

During labor and birth there is simultaneous control: you and nature are working together. Nature is leading, your mind and body are accepting the lead. You are controlling your mind and with it, your body's response.

It's a synergistic relationship with great results!

To have a visual image of the difference between accepting a situation and resisting a situation, let's look at Alan Watt's example from his book "Wisdom of Insecurity." Picture two trees, the willow tree and the pine tree. In a snowstorm, the unyielding branches of the pine tree accumulate snow until they crack. The springy boughs of the willow tree bend under the weight, drop the snow, and bounce back again.

Your mind has the same powers.

During each contraction accept what is happening, get through it however you can, let it go, and rest for the next one.

Focus on the Present Moment

If you find yourself thinking ahead and dreading each upcoming contraction or wondering how much longer labor will last or how much longer you can handle the pain, you are not in the present moment.

If you find yourself obsessing over your current dilation, or the rate of it over the past few hours, or lamenting over how long you've been laboring up to this point, you are not in the present moment.

Change your focus to the present moment, the current contraction; that's all there is.

There is no past and there is no future; there is only now. **There is only the current contraction**. Deal with each contraction as it comes, without judging the past or anticipating the future.

Sharing My Story

This advice was very helpful for me; not once was I thinking ahead. I was only concentrating on relaxing my body and breathing down the energy through each contraction.

Sharing Stories: Staying Present

"Let go of your fear, and give in to the moment. I never felt scared or frightened by what my body was doing or what I was feeling. It was a terrible pain, hurt like hell, but each contraction ended and it was OK. You just gear up for the next one. Just take one at a time and know it's not forever." – Courtney

"I used a lot of self-talk, taking each contraction one at a time. I tried to be in the moment and not think too far ahead....I was very present through it all. I was glad I let my body do its thing. I was amazed at the process and what we can do if we don't fight and let it happen." – Bonnie

"I also turned around all clocks so I had no idea how much time had passed." – Kristen

Focus on Breathing

The best way to divert your focus away from pain is to focus on breathing.

The best way to focus on accepting labor and being in the present moment is to focus on breathing.

Sharing Stories: Breathing

"[Most important during labor was] breathing. Warm bath. Moving around. Counter pressure on my lower back during contractions. Positive encouragement from everyone in the room. Visualizing my baby and telling myself that she will get here quicker and safer if I can get through the pain. Taking one contraction at a time. BREATHING. Did I already say that?" – Karen H.

"[Most helpful during labor was] doing my own thing and breathing at my own pace with eyes closed." – Stephanie

"[Most helpful during labor was] breathing, staying relaxed, and my doula/friend support. – Nina

Paradoxes of Vulnerability

Feels weak, but is strong.
Feels like loss of control, but in control of mind.

"And so you touch this limit, something happens and you suddenly can go a little bit further. With your mind power, your determination, your instinct, and the experience as well, you can fly very high." – Ayrton Senna

CHAPTER 8
STAY HYDRATED AND NOURISHED

"The question isn't who is going to let me; it's who is going to stop me." – Ayn Rand

Labor is hard work and can take many hours. Just as with any other activity that requires strength and endurance, your body needs to be hydrated and fueled during labor. The right sustenance can give you the energy to continue your hard work through to the end, so you can have the natural birth of your dreams!

Your body will let you know what kind of hydration and nutrition it may (or may not) need. Always listen to and trust your body. There may be times you don't feel like eating or drinking anything. It is important to have the option, to have a choice.

If you are thirsty, drink. If you are hungry, eat.

Not being allowed to eat and drink during labor can take away a sense of control. Thirst is a source of discomfort during labor and remaining comfortable is important for having a natural birth. Water is a good choice, as are fruit juices, electrolyte drinks, and teas.

If you do eat, choose food that is easy to digest so your body can use its resources for labor. Small bites of snack food are good, such as soft fruit, yogurt, or broth.

A related piece of advice is to urinate often during labor; it will help you stay comfortable and it keeps labor moving along. Reminding you to stay hydrated and use the bathroom is a good job for your support person.

Sharing My Story

I didn't feel like eating much during labor with my first child; I tried eating lunch but felt nauseous. Once we got to the birth center I took a few bites of an apple, but it tasted way too sweet so I didn't eat anything else. My body was saying no to food, but yes to hydration. I drank water and an electrolyte solution during labor. (During, and after, the birth of our daughter I sipped on coconut water.)

Just a few hours after our son was born, the apple was still sitting on the table and I took a bite of it. I was surprised to discover that it tasted normal again, and delicious. The highly sweet taste during labor was probably my body's way of telling me I didn't need it at the time.

Staying Hydrated in the Hospital

Many (or most) laboring women are hooked up to an IV for fluids instead of being allowed to drink. However, studies show there is no evidence of harm from eating and drinking during labor. Thus, there is no justification for the restriction of fluids and food in labor for women at low risk of complications.

Sharing a Story

A friend who birthed all four of her children naturally in a hospital intentionally eats a good meal right before she heads to the hospital, knowing she won't be allowed to eat anything once she gets there.

CHAPTER 9
COMFORT AND COPING TECHNIQUES

"Perseverance is the hard work you do after you get tired of doing the hard work you already did." – Aristotle

Change the Way You View the Pain

Think of the pain you feel during labor as nature's way to encourage you to seek comfort. One laboring position may feel great for a while and then you may need to find a different one. Your body sends signals for you to respond to. By accepting nature's cues and responding to what you feel, you are working together to help the baby rotate and descend, thus helping labor progress.

Sharing Stories: How to View the Pain

"Trust your body. Know that the pain you feel is a pain that passes so quickly. It is a 'good' pain." – Andrea

"It's not painful as long as you can relax and breathe with each contraction. It's only temporary and so worth it." – Abbey

"I focused on what my body was doing instead of how it was feeling." – Talitha

Comfort and Coping Techniques

The more **confident** you are that you will be able to cope, the **less pain** you will feel. Hopefully knowing the many techniques that are available will be one part of increasing your confidence.

Make sure your partner and care provider are aware of these different comfort and coping techniques and ideas so they can suggest them to you. You will be focused on the present moment and probably not able to think of the list.

To help you visualize the techniques mentioned below, here is a link to a free download created by Penny Simkin, which includes drawings and descriptions of ways to find comfort during labor. (childbirthconnection.org/pdfs/comfort-in-labor-simkin.pdf)

Mental Techniques

** Meditation and Prayer: Sit in silence while focusing on your breathing. Recite a helpful or meaningful prayer.

** Mantras and Affirmations: Repeat a mantra to yourself during each contraction, synchronized with your breathing, such as, "Inhale and open. Exhale and open more." or "My body is created to do this. I have nothing to fear." It may also be helpful if your support person says your prayers, mantras, or affirmations to you while you focus on breathing.

** Visualization: Picture yourself as a supple willow tree, bending as the snow accumulates, dropping it, and bouncing back again. Picture each contraction as a wave; let the wave come and ride it until it's over. Picture yourself as a strong, capable animal giving birth. Visualize your baby moving down the birth canal. Visualize your cervix opening. Visualize a flower opening or the sun rising.

These visualizations can be made into mantras to be repeated, such as "I am opening so much." or "My body opens easily." or "Open, open, open." or "My mind quiets. My body opens. My baby descends."

** Hypnosis: If you have taken any hypnosis-for-childbirth classes, you will know the techniques involved in entering a state of hypnosis.

Sensory Techniques

** Smell: Essential oils are a good way to help cover any hospital smells you may not like. (Several drops on a cotton ball placed in a jar or baggie might be helpful.)

** Sound: Listening to calm, soothing, and familiar music can help maintain a relaxed body and atmosphere. A white noise machine may be a good option, especially to conceal hospital noises. Sometimes you may also want no sounds at all, just soft voices.

** Sight: Having a visual focus point may help some women, such as an interesting lava lamp, photo frame with rotating photos, a few actual photos to hold, a picture of a beautiful nature scene, or some affirmations placed on the wall.

** Touch: Activate sensors in your fingertips by moving your fingertips in circles on the sheet or a pleasing fabric, fingering soft textures like velvet or stuffed animals, or feeling your partner's face.

Physical Techniques

** Breathing: Use conscious, slow breathing through the contractions. Exhale like you mean it, strong and controlled, like you are pushing the energy/pain out of your body with your breath.

** Vocalizing: A natural and instinctual way of coping with labor, vocalizing in low-pitched tones releases the energy from your body. Any audible noises can be helpful, including moaning, groaning, chanting, sighing, humming, and singing. Low-pitched noises are made with a relaxed throat, jaw, and mouth. High-pitched tones, such as screaming or screeching, can indicate panic and may prevent progress.

** Hydrotherapy: Take a shower; or sit on a chair or birth ball in the shower and spray warm water on your belly or back. Later in labor, perhaps when 5-6cm+ dilation, you may want to sit in a tub of warm water. (Sitting in warm water too early can stall labor.)

** Change positions: Walk around. Sit on a birth ball (sit up, rock, bounce gently, or lean forward with arms on a bed). Be on your hands and knees. Squat. Stand and slow dance or sway with the support of your partner. Find a position that feels good; change your position often or as you feel.

** Acupressure: There are several acupressure points on the body; foot, hands, ankles, buttocks, shoulder. For information about the specific acupressure point, ask your acupuncturist or search online.

** Hot/cold packs: Having something ready to help with temperature changes that can occur at different stages of labor can be helpful. Personal fans can be nice for this, too.

** Massage: Using natural massage oils, a massage can help mom relax. There are a couple of areas on the body to massage that feels great during labor such as thighs and feet.

** Counter-pressure: For back labor, having someone apply counter-pressure can really help. A sock filled with a couple tennis balls is a good tool for this.

** Touch: Sometimes the laboring mom does not want a massage but touch might be a preferred alternative. A simple touch on an area that is tense (such as the jaw, arm, leg) might provide comfort and a reminder to relax. Activate sensors in the palms, soles of feet, and lips by having your partner hold your hand, rub your feet, or kiss you.

Sharing My Story

When my vocalization increased in intensity and volume later in labor, it sounded like deep and primal moaning, instead of high-pitched anxiety. I remember apologizing to my midwives during my labors for the loud noises I was making. Knowing that vocalizing is a normal and important part of labor, they always reassured me by saying, "You weren't that loud." or

"You just make whatever noises you need to make."

My throat was sore for a day and a half after my son's birth from all the vocalizing I did.

Sharing My Story

During labor with our first child, for many contractions I leaned forward into my husband's palm which rested on my forehead. Feeling his hand there provided me stability, safety, comfort, and routine.

During labor with our second child, my husband placed his hand on my lower back (as I leaned forward) or on my arm. There was no motion involved, so it wasn't a massage, but the steady touch that was available for every contraction was a welcome focal point and calming mechanism. It helped me to know I wasn't doing this alone.

Sharing Stories: Coping With Labor Pain

"I think being free to roam the room and find the most comfortable positions was the most helpful. If something worked, I would just keep doing it until it no longer worked." – Abbey

"I would labor in a warm shower and use the birthing ball to help open my pelvis. I also played music to help 'carry me away' during intense contractions." – Tatiana

"[Most helpful during labor was] staying relaxed moving around. It also helped that out of my 14-hour labor it didn't really get intense until the last hour." – Melanie

"[Most helpful during labor was] lots of birth positions, breathing, and being in a tub." – Emily

"I instinctively went into a light hypnotic state and focused well. I had practiced meditation from my teens onward, and it was easy for me to go inwards." – Margaret

"[Most helpful during labor was] getting into comfortable positions and moving." – Annette

"[Most helpful during labor was] being left alone to cope as I saw fit. Getting in the water and just riding each wave." – Fonda

"[Most helpful during labor was] focusing on the outcome—a baby born with all the benefits of natural hormones, going through the birth canal, an alert momma." – Arusi

Help Me Help You: Tips for Your Birth Partner

"For birth companions to simply be, to do nothing when nothing is all there is to be done, to offer support without judgement, guidance without attachment, love without conditions—that is perhaps the greatest challenge and the greatest gift." – Vicki Chan, Midwife

During pregnancy it is helpful to discover ways that your partner can support you during labor. Having different ways to offer **reminders and reassurance** is important. It is also important for your partner to have compassion for you in labor and not fear your labor pain.

Your partner can offer **reminders**:

** To make low-toned noises during contractions to help release the energy.

** To say "yes" to each contraction, allowing it to happen instead of fighting it.

** About your reasons for wanting a natural birth.

** About your baby: "Each contraction is bringing you closer to holding your baby in your arms" or "Our baby is so excited to meet you soon" or "Our baby feels your love right now" or "Breathe down your energy to our baby."

** By speaking words of love, such as: "I love you," "You're amazing," "You're really doing it," and "I'm so proud of you." Find whatever words might work for you personally and make a list for your partner.

** About your mantras, visualizations, and prayers, either saying them to you as you breathe through a contraction, or reminding you of ones you can say to yourself.

Your partner can offer **reassurance**:

** About anything that might make you feel self-conscious. If or when bodily fluids or sounds appear, your partner can reassure you that it's no big deal and completely normal.

** By acknowledging your feelings. Most of us want empathy during labor. Admit that pain is pain; don't pretend it's not. Your partner can empathize with the pain, and then respond with encouragement. "This hurts so much" can be met with "It's really painful. But you are stronger than this is hard."

** About your strength. "I can't do this anymore" can be met with "You are doing it and you are doing wonderfully."

If there ever comes a time when your partner doesn't know how to offer support, remind him to love you through it. Comfort, reassurance, patience, and love are the best labor companions.

Sharing Stories: Support and Reassurance During Labor

"*After 32 hours of very hard labor we were at a point where I was talking about going to the hospital and 'giving up' essentially. I overheard my midwife talking with my mom and she said, 'If I know her, then she will keep doing it. She wants this.' Hearing her faith in me, and saying how it was what I wanted, reaffirmed my desire to keep going and that simple comment gave me the strength to keep going.*" – Marissa

"*[Most helpful during labor was] my husband. He knew how important it was to me. When I would start to cave he would remind me how much I wanted a natural birth and would encourage me.*" – Kayla

"*[Most helpful during labor was] having the support of my husband and midwives. Being open about how I was feeling and my fears and anxieties. By verbalizing those feelings as they came up, I was able to work through them to get to a place of strength again. I found I cycled through feeling fearful and unsure, to strong and determined. My husband especially helped me through this by being unwavering in his confidence in me. This process was far more important than any of the practical things that helped me, like warm water, counter pressure, or having a water birth." – Leah*

"[Most helpful during labor was] stubborn resolve and a supportive partner and birth team making sure I was hydrated and as comfortable as possible." – Angela

"It's easier if you are with people who know your wishes and also can provide suggestions, massage, etc." – Jenny

"Knowing it would be over soon kept me confident and having at least one person who understood and was supportive of what I wanted." – Christina

"Have a doula or other support person with you to make suggestions during labor such as take a drink of water or get on the birthing ball or try a certain technique....Also, have that person remind you every once in a while of why you are there, doing what you're doing; soon you will hold a baby in your arms, and that all the pain is for a reason." – Chenae

Comfort Techniques in a Hospital

Hospital policies will vary on what techniques may be used for coping with pain during a birth. Ask ahead of time so you know what items they have available, such as birth balls, showers, tubs for laboring, or a squatting rack.

"We are made to do this work and it's not easy...I would say that pain is part of the glory, or the tremendous mystery of life. And that if anything, it's a kind of privilege to stand so close to such an incredible miracle." – Simone in Klasson

CHAPTER 10
BIRTH IN A POSITION YOU CHOOSE

"Except for being hanged by the feet, the supine position is the worst conceivable position for labor and delivery." – Roberto Caldeyro-Barcia, past president of the International Federation of Obstetricians and Gynecologists

With your freedom to move according to how you feel during a natural childbirth, you will probably be in a variety of positions throughout your labor. Likewise, when it's time to push your baby out you will instinctively know which position feels good to you at that time.

Birthing in a position you choose validates your body's natural inclinations for movement and position and supports your autonomy in the process.

Ideal Birth Positions

"An ideal birth position allows the mother's sacrum and coccyx the freedom to rotate backward, the rest of the pelvis room to open to optimal dimensions to allow for birth, and contractions to remain strong and close together." – Anne Frye, Holistic Midwifery

Evidence supports the use of upright and side-lying positions as safer and healthier for mom and baby, with results of shorter pushing time, fewer forceps or vacuum births, fewer episiotomies, less severe pain, and fewer abnormal fetal heart rate patterns. Positions other than on your back include:

** Hands and knees: This position is helpful for turning a posterior baby, back labor, and birthing a large baby.

** Side-lying: This position is good in the latter stages of labor and for a long labor as it promotes full body rest and relaxation. This is also a good pushing position for fast labors as well as for first-time moms since the baby comes out a bit slower, allowing the perineum time to stretch and hopefully avoid tearing.

** Squatting: Squatting opens up the pelvis and helps align baby for optimal birth position. You may want to hold on to a squatting bar, towel, or your partner for balance.

** Sitting: Sitting positions allow gravity to work, as well as aid in relaxation. They are also beneficial because the mother's weight is supported without putting pressure on the perineum. You could try sitting on the thighs of your partner or on a birth chair to aid this position. Sitting positions are NOT the same as semi-sitting (reclining) positions.

** Vertical or standing: Upright positions use gravity to assist in the birth, helping the baby drop into the pelvis and find a good position. You can stand and lean forward onto a counter or your partner for support.

Avoid Supine/Lithotomy Position

The supine/lithotomy (flat-on-back) position is the most commonly used position in vaginal births in hospitals (68%); a close second is the reclining (or semi-sitting) position (23%). However, they are not optimal positions for birth and are used mostly for the convenience of the hospital staff.

There are several disadvantages of birthing on your back:
** More painful than other positions
** Creates narrowest pelvic opening
** Restricts the movement of the coccyx (tailbone) which can make it harder for baby's head to come out
** Reduces blood flow to the baby

Birth Positions in a Hospital

It is possible to birth in a position of your choice at a hospital, although this is a location where you may run into some resistance. Hospital policy as well as the opinions, preferences, and experience of the staff will vary. Freedom of movement during pushing is another reason to request intermittent fetal monitoring, instead of continuous EFM.

Since you won't have an epidural you will be able to move and change positions. If you pick your position and are already pushing when the doctor appears, they may just go with the flow and support you.

Sharing My Story

During my first pregnancy, I was sure I would choose some sort of upright position for pushing, wanting to take full advantage of gravity. I was surprised when I ended up in the side-lying position for pushing with both of my births. I pushed for 30 minutes with my son and for 20 minutes with my daughter. It was a comfortable position for me. I did not tear with either birth.

Sharing a Story

When friend of mine arrived at the hospital in labor, a nurse had her lie down on the bed to check her cervix, which was fully dilated to 10cm. Lying on the bed was too uncomfortable so when the exam was over, she got up to walk around and the nurse suggested she lean against the counter. Soon the doctor arrived, joking about it being so early in the morning he hadn't even had his coffee yet. The nurse asked him if he'd ever delivered a baby standing up, and he joked that he'd "tried to make a few that way, but we've come this far so why not give it a shot."

"There is no way out of the experience except through it, because it is not really your experience at all but the baby's. Your body is the child's instrument of birth." – Penelope Leach

CHAPTER 11
PUSH INSTINCTIVELY

"There is power that comes to women when they give birth. They don't ask for it, it simply invades them. Accumulates like clouds on the horizon and passes through, carrying the child with it." – Sheryl Feldman

A common worry about natural childbirth is the pain related to the pushing phase. If you ask around you will hear varying responses about how pushing feels, from very painful to pain free. There could be many reasons for this, but choosing an effective (non-supine) position will go a long way to reducing pain during the pushing phase, as discussed previously.

Women instinctively know how to push, so I would recommend following your body's natural urge as the baby moves down the birth canal. It may mean spontaneous pushing, which is pushing when and how much your body feels like pushing. It may mean exhale pushing, which is like a gentle, controlled deep breath with a purposeful exhale.

The opposite (directed pushing) is associated with the baby receiving less oxygen as well as with an increased risk of pelvic floor dysfunction.

Remember, by continually inhaling and exhaling you will keep oxygen flowing to your baby. Since you will not be medicated you will be able to feel what your body needs you to do.

Crowning

For both of my births crowning did hurt a bit, but it was a stinging sensation and it didn't last long at all. (If I had to guess strictly from memory, I would say it lasted about 10-15 seconds.) Both times my midwife asked me to stop pushing for a moment, so that the baby could crown nice and slowly, to avoid tearing.

Pushing Support

There are a couple ways to help be more comfortable during the pushing phase:
  ** Follow your body's signals
  ** Have your caregiver apply perineal support, perhaps applying a warm compress
  ** Birth in a side-lying position

Sharing Stories: Pushing

My friend Juliana shared how helpful it was to be able to take a few breaths from an oxygen mask between pushes. Squatting on the hospital bed while she pushed, she would lean back against the raised bed where the mask was laying, take a few breaths, and be ready to push again. She said it helped give her energy to keep pushing.

"When I had to push I would envision my baby coming down the birth canal with each contraction/push, which helped me to stay somewhat relaxed, especially when he/she began to crown… It was amazing to feel my baby descend down. I felt better connected to each of my children; we did it together." – Tatiana

"I was pretty stunned by how much it hurt (crowning/pushing)." – Lauren

"My first was a 27-hour labor with three hours of pushing out a compound-presentation large-headed baby (hand by head)…I told my husband two hours post-birth that I couldn't wait to do it again!" – Stacy

Sharing My Story: Breathing Baby Out/Exhale Pushing

For my son's birth, I pushed by breathing down through the contractions. In between contractions I rested. I didn't feel like I was pushing, the contractions were doing most of the work. I was breathing deep belly breaths. I felt like I breathed my baby out, instead of pushed him out.

With each push, especially closer to birth, I could feel the baby move down. And when the contraction stopped and I stopped pushing, he would retract a little. With each push, he came farther out, and then would retract. Each push means more progress, almost like "two steps forward, one step back."

Once my son's head was showing, our midwife asked if I wanted to touch it. I did and it was amazing! It gave me an adrenaline rush to finish, knowing I was so close! It was very powerful emotionally to have the connection between what I was feeling in my belly and bottom and what I was feeling with my hand.

Sharing My Story: Spontaneous Pushing

With my daughter, pushing didn't feel as slow and controlled as it did with my son. I pushed harder and was so focused on pushing, pushing, pushing, that my midwife (thankfully) would remind me to stop pushing when the contraction ended, advising me to save my strength.

That brings up another point: In this stage of labor you are probably in a different mental state, in a zone and focused. In such a state you are highly susceptible to suggestions. This is why it's of the utmost importance that you trust everyone around you to only give suggestions that you would agree with if you were in a rational mind. I trusted my midwife and knew that if she said to take a break, I should take a break.

After my water broke (10 minutes before she was born) I felt the sensation of her sliding down, closer to coming out. She felt really small and it was an incredible sensation, making me think she was just going to slide right out!

"Everything is hard before it is easy." – Johann Wolfgang von Goethe

CHAPTER 12
AFTER YOUR NATURAL BIRTH

"The instant of birth is exquisite. Pain and joy are one at this moment. Ever after, the dim recollection is so sweet that we speak to our children with a gratitude they never understand." – *Madline Tiger*

Congratulations! Your baby is here and you achieved the natural birth of your dreams!

You may experience the surge of hormones that occurs at the end of a natural birth, creating a great euphoric state. Right after both my births, I was making such a noise you couldn't tell if I was laughing or crying. I reassured everyone that I was completely thrilled!

Moments After Birth

Here are a few things you may want to do in the first few minutes, hours, and days after your natural birth.

** **Skin to skin:** Immediately after birth, have your baby placed on your belly for some wonderful skin-to-skin contact.

** **Keep baby in your arms:** Take these first few minutes and hours to bond with your baby.

** **Breastfeed:** Initiate breastfeeding within the first hour or two of birth. Hopefully your care providers help you get a good start. Even though breastfeeding is a natural extension of birth that doesn't mean it will always be an easy road. Be prepared to ask for help at any point along the journey, but especially at the beginning. Have the number of a good lactation consultant ready and call if you need help.

** **Get up and walk:** Once your care provider has given you the go-ahead, you can get up and walk fairly soon after birth. Within the first hour or two I was given the task of trying to use the bathroom, which required a short walk across the room.

** **Shower:** Although baths may have to wait, your care provider will let you know when it is okay for you to take a shower.

** **Rest and Recover:** Birth is hard work and now is the time to rest and recover. It was hard for me to stay in bed like I was advised because I felt so great. Sure I was sore, but I was definitely able to walk around and do things. Looking back, I wish I would have taken advantage of those first few days and just napped and rested as much as I could, with my new baby right beside me.

** **Babymoon:** I recommend keeping visitors and any other socializing to a minimum in the first few weeks. This is your special time to rest and connect with your new baby. Unless you know for sure that a guest will be "low maintenance" and be there to help you or to drop off a meal, give yourself a couple weeks to figure things out before welcoming a parade of visitors that you need to entertain.

** **Write your birth story:** In order to remember all the little details I recommend writing your birth story within a week of the birth. (Trust me, as time goes by you will forget the little details.) It doesn't have to be fancy; just get the facts down on paper or in a word processing document. Birth stories are treasures for you and for your children. Also, have your partner write a birth story from their perspective. My husband wrote one after our son was born and it was so touching to read the story from his point of view.

** **Share your birth story:** When you talk to people, share your story of birth. Whenever anyone asks who delivered your baby, look them in the eye, smile, and proudly say, "I did."

Sharing Stories: After a Natural Birth

"When my baby came out, I couldn't believe it was over. Just like that. There he was. It was amazing. I was exhausted and overwhelmed because just like that you become a mom, learn to nurse. I was released four hours later so very tired and sore. I had been up for 36 hours. It's not easy, but it's worth it." – Courtney

"After having a natural birth with my first child, I knew that I could do it again. The recovery was fast, and the most rewarding part was feeling that relief and happiness once the baby came out and I was able to hold him. I now have three kids, all natural births. No regrets. I would not numb the experience by having an epidural." – Julia

"[I felt] proud of myself, excited to do it again, thought it wasn't as bad as I had thought it could have been (was 17 hours long too!)" – Emily

"As soon as the baby was out, I felt like super woman and the pain was gone completely. My recovery was very fast and less than an hour after giving birth I walked to

my recovery room on my own." – Malisa

"*My baby started breastfeeding within an hour of her birth which I contribute to not having any drugs during her birth (I have no scientific info to back this up—just my instincts). My first struggled to breastfeed for the first 2-4 weeks of his life. Don't get me wrong, I was in pain (2nd-degree tear) but I was in pain after my first, too (3rd-degree tear). It felt so good to do what naturally felt right. I felt like I gave my baby a gift."* – Karen H.

"*Initially I felt spent and even traumatized. It was extremely hard to give birth to my daughter and I experienced things (emotions) I did not expect, so there was surprise too. But I also felt so proud of myself and elated. My body felt excellent afterward. Gee, I felt so good! I was up walking around almost straight away. Some friends who had not had much experience with natural birth commented on how great I looked afterwards. I loved hearing that. A few weeks later I had processed the experience more fully and began to see just how wonderful the experience was. I can't wait to do it again!"* – Leah

"*I recovered quite quickly. The first couple days were a high of hormones and emotions and I felt great (if tired). About days 3-6 I felt pretty delicate and wiped out, then after that I had to force myself to rest because I felt fine and wanted to be up and active. There was always a feeling of awe about what I just accomplished as well."* – Jamie

"*[I felt] powerful, like I could scale a 10-story building. We are done having children, but I am truly sad that I will never get to give birth again. Nothing is as empowering as having a natural birth. Since I am a runner along with being a yogi, I often say that I feel like giving birth is like running your best race ever with your best friend and getting the ultimate prize."* – Katie

I CAN AND I WILL

PART 3: MY NATURAL BIRTH STORIES

"So the question remains. Is childbirth painful? Yes. It can be, along with a thousand amazing sensations for which we have yet to find adequate language. Every birth is different, and every woman's experience and telling of her story will be unique." – Marcie Macari

It's important to surround yourself with as many natural birth stories as you can. This is how it becomes normal to you. To start you off, I'd like to share my two natural birth stories.

I CAN AND I WILL

CHAPTER 13
BIRTH STORY OF OUR SON, BIRTH CENTER BIRTH, MARCH 2007

The night before my son was born, I went to bed about 10:30 p.m. but didn't fall asleep until midnight. I woke up at 2 a.m. with a really bad back ache, which kept me from being comfortable enough to sleep. The pain went away about 3 a.m., but then I had other aches and pains which continued for another hour.

At 4 a.m., as I was trying to fall asleep, I felt a slight pain in my low belly and then it went away. A few minutes later it came back, and then it went away. My thought was "I think those are contractions." I tried to go to sleep, but they were already kind of painful and pretty close together. I'm not sure how long I laid there (maybe an hour or so) but it was obvious that I wasn't going to be able to sleep. I got up and went to the bathroom and saw some pink on the tissue. Wow, I know what this means. I think I am in labor!

My husband stirred at this point and I said I was going to go lie on the couch and that I am going to have your son today. He mumbled something and went back to sleep.

I decided to lie on the couch and listen to my Hypnobabies CDs. I was sure that I could remove the pain because I was very good about doing all the required lessons for the class. I believed it would work and I would feel no pain. So I started my CDs, turned my light switch off, and went into hypnosis waiting for my anesthesia to work (Hypnobabies terms). I was so disappointed when it didn't work for me; I felt a lot of pain. My contractions started out about five minutes apart. I always thought labor would start more gradually; 20 minutes apart, then 15, then 10, etc. Not for me. No rest for me.

I called the birthing center about 9:15 a.m. or so to give them a heads up. Our midwife said I didn't need to start timing the contractions quite yet. She also said, "It sounds like you might have a baby today or tomorrow."

I lay on the couch for a while, not sure how long. I was just deep breathing and trying to relax and not tense up, for which I can thank Hypnobabies. I did get pretty anxious about how I would handle the day without my anesthesia (Hypnobabies term) like I had planned. I sent a frantic email to my Hypnobabies email group asking what I could do. I was crying as I wrote that email.

From the computer as I typed that email, I looked outside and saw my husband putting mulch in the flower beds. That was surreal. I was feeling what I was feeling and he was doing mulch. (I did tell him he should do what he needs to do early on because he might not be able to do it later.)

I then took a shower, taking care to shave my legs really well. :) I tried to eat lunch but just couldn't stomach it.

We then started timing the contractions and noticed they were about 2-3 minutes apart and 45-65 seconds long. They were getting worse. So I get into the bathroom to do the important stuff—like put on makeup and curl my hair. That took a long time because the contractions were so strong that I would need to stop what I was doing and put my head into my husband's palm to focus.

Some of the contractions were making me feel really nauseous towards the end. I made myself vomit. I thought that was another sign I was getting close, maybe even in transition. I called the birth center and our midwife said we could come in and get checked.

It took a long time to get all our stuff gathered. I had already packed my bag, but we needed to get all the bags and food and gear together. The car ride to the birthing center should only take about 10 minutes, but it seemed longer than that. We hit every light we could. Contractions in a moving vehicle are no fun, especially when going over bumps in the road.

We arrived about 3 p.m. and then our midwife checked me between contractions and announced I was "almost 4." "What?? That's all?" I said. She said it was pretty good, those are the hardest ones. She said we could either go home to labor there, or we could walk around the gardens for an hour and she would check me again. We opted to do the latter, as there was no way I was getting in that car again.

We walked and walked and walked in that garden. During each contraction, I would hug Dave and lean into him and he would say things like "Relax," "Peace," "Release the energy." Those words were perfect to hear. I tried to just relax and not let my body tense up. I think I did that pretty well.

We came in after the hour and she checked me again. I can't remember her exact words but I think she said I was a "strong 4" or a "4+," something like that. She said that was good progress for an hour and we were allowed to stay. This was about 4:15 p.m. She helped me up the stairs while Dave went to get our stuff out of the car. We didn't make it very far up the stairs in that time.

She suggested I sit on the birth ball or take a shower. I opted to start on the birth ball. I sat on it and leaned forward onto the bed. I listened to a Hypnobabies CD (can't remember which one). I sat on the birth ball for about an hour (until about 5:30).

Then I got into the shower. I sat on a chair and held the sprayer to my belly. That felt nice! I sat in there for about a half hour, until 6:15 or so. I put on my shorts and then our midwife suggested I walk around for a while. I was going to, but then felt too tired and said I just wanted to lie down for a while. That would end up being the last position I was in the rest of the night.

The contractions started getting worse, and when I mentioned it to her she said, "They are supposed to." I started feeling kind of grunty with them, not necessarily pushy. And I started to be quite vocal, releasing the energy with low-pitched moans and such noises; really primal. That surprised me. I didn't think I would be so loud. But our midwife and Dave both assured me I wasn't that loud and that it was normal to vocalize.

After a while of feeling grunty, almost pushy during the contractions, I felt a goosh and said "Uh oh, my water." My water had just broken! Our midwife checked the baby's heartbeat again, since she said they sometimes get stressed out when the water breaks. But it was still strong (as it had been each time she checked before). She checked me after my water broke (around 7 p.m.) and said I was at 9cm—to the surprise of all of us! Wow, almost there already!

After almost an hour of deep, loud sounds and breathing down the energy, she checked me again. She said something like "no more cervix" and I asked "10?" and she said "Yes, 10." This was approximately 8 p.m.

I was thinking I might have that "rest and be thankful" phase that I had read about, but no, contractions kept going. I felt like my body was leading and I was just following along with a bit of pushing to help out. It was so surreal to feel the little bulge when I pushed. It didn't feel like a baby's head because it felt small, not big.

As the pushes went on, I could feel him coming farther and farther out, and then feel him retracting back in. I remember our midwife pointing out that each time, he retracted less and less. Dave got to look down and see hair on his head. Our midwife asked if I wanted to feel his head. I was a bit scared to, so didn't say anything. Several minutes later she asked again and I touched his head and said "my baby"—what a wonderful moment!

I kept pushing with the contractions and resting in between. At one point she said to not push so hard, I think he was almost crowning. I think when he was crowning, I felt a bit of stinging and think I whimpered. Our midwife said some words of encouragement, I can't remember what exactly. I do remember her saying that with the next push our baby would be born. I pushed and then the head came out. Then another push and I felt the body just slide right out. He's here! Our son was born at 8:36 p.m.

She placed him on my belly and I just started crying, almost hysterically I was so overjoyed. I can't remember what I said exactly. He was just so beautiful! I couldn't believe how clean he was, no blood or guck on him at all. I looked over at Dave and saw tears on his face.

When the cord stopped pulsing, Dave cut it. Our son was right on my belly when they did this. They weighed him and announced 8 lbs 0.5 oz, bigger than they thought he would be.

I did not think I would birth in a side-lying position; I always thought I wanted gravity to help me out. But it was easy. Our midwife said it might help first-time moms to not tear. And I didn't, which is great!

My throat was sore for about a day and a half afterwards, from all my "vocalizing."

Having a natural childbirth was tough, but absolutely worth it to me. I would do it again in a heartbeat. I loved how great I felt immediately afterward. I loved birthing in a birth center and the care of a midwife. It was the perfect atmosphere for all of us and I am so grateful for this amazing experience.

Here is a photo of our new family, just minutes after our son was born.

We left the birth center about 1:30 a.m., driving home on a quiet and foggy night.

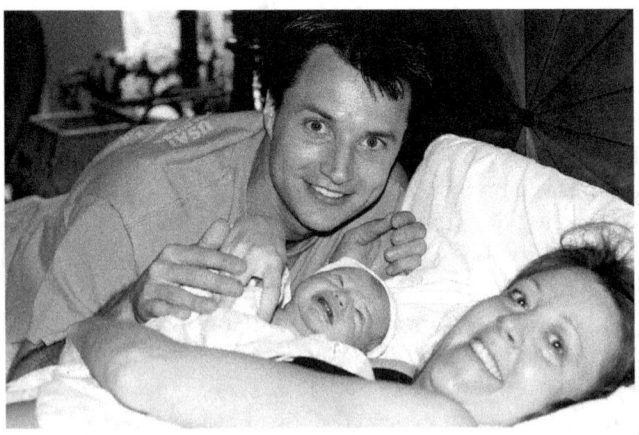

CHAPTER 14
BIRTH STORY OF OUR DAUGHTER, HOME BIRTH, SEPTEMBER 2011

On Tuesday September 6, my due date, I started having intense Braxton Hicks contractions that slowly became more painful throughout the day. When I went to bed at 10 p.m., they became full-blown, intense contractions that came every 20 minutes—all night long. They were so intense that I had a hard time relaxing to the end of one. They weren't close enough to bring a baby, but were strong enough to keep me awake all night. About 7 a.m. they died down and went away for a while.

Throughout the day Wednesday I had contractions on and off; sometimes 20 minutes apart, sometimes 30-45 minutes apart. Early Wednesday evening I became weepy and frustrated, not knowing what was happening with all these spaced-apart contractions. I knew my body was getting ready, but I wasn't prepared for the randomness of contractions over such a long period of time. I felt like I needed to talk to someone so about 7:30 p.m. I called the midwife on call.

I told her we weren't ready for her to come yet, but asked if she could give me pep talk. She was great talking to me, said I sounded sleep-deprived, and offered some suggestions. One of her suggestions was to take a bath. She said it might reset me and perhaps help me sleep. She said she thought she'd be hearing from us later that night (which I really didn't believe). I said I didn't want an all-nighter birth and she said babies just come when they do.

I felt better after talking to her and decided to take a bath. I was in the bath from 8-8:30 p.m. It felt great but I was surprised that it didn't take away all the pain from the several contractions I had while in the tub.

About 9 p.m. I noticed that the contractions were coming closer together and I needed Dave with me during them. (Before this I was able to handle them by myself.) Dave was going back and forth between me and Griffin, trying to help me while he was trying to put Griffin to bed. But Griffin just said "I want to see what you guys are doing!"

So we decided that I needed to move out of our bathroom, since Griffin was trying to go to sleep in our bed. I went to Griffin's room to labor. Once Dave got him to bed he joined me. The contractions were so close together that at 10 p.m. we thought we better start timing them. We saw right away that they were about 2:20 apart and lasting from 45-60 seconds. After timing them for 15 minutes, and seeing they were consistently this far apart, we decided we better call our midwife back.

Dave called her about 10:15 p.m. and she said she'd be here in about 30 minutes. Dave then called the birth photographer. I heard her say she might wait until the midwife got to the house and checked me. Then a contraction started and she must have heard me because I heard her say "Is that Wendy? I'm on my way."

I didn't want to birth in Griffin's room so we moved back to our bathroom. Griffin was asleep in our bed by now. Dave laughed when I said I needed to change clothes since I didn't want to wear what I was wearing (pajamas). He laughed even harder when I started putting makeup on in between contractions. Hey, there are going to be pictures taken, I better look half-way decent in them! (In my defense, I didn't curl my hair this time, although the thought did cross my mind.)

Our midwife arrived about 10:45 p.m. and immediately started getting my IV antibiotics ready. Once it was in she stood there and held the bag until it was empty. The birth assistant arrived shortly after that, and not too much later, the birth photographer arrived.

Shortly after our midwife arrived, Dave moved Griffin out of our room and onto the floor of the living room. I continued to labor in our bathroom, leaning over the counter for each contraction while Dave would say "breathe and release."

I did try laying on the bed on my left side for a few contractions but that didn't feel great so back to standing in the bathroom. I was trying so hard not to squeeze and push during the contractions because I didn't want my water to break, knowing that the longer it stayed intact the more protection for the baby. At one point our midwife mentioned that I was sounding "pushy." I didn't think much of it at the time, besides agreeing with her, but I wonder if I was fully dilated and actually ready to push? My cervix was never checked so I don't know how dilated I was at any given time.

I felt panicky during the contractions, which was surprising to me; maybe because of how fast and intense it was, maybe because I couldn't relax through them (like I did during Griffin's birth). I felt kind of out of control which was not how I wanted it to be.

Our midwife asked if I wanted to see what happened on the bed and I remember not wanting to do that for some reason. I did keep saying I felt like I had to go to the bathroom so I tried one time. Our midwife thought that was the baby I was feeling, even though I didn't think it was. I finally agreed to lie on the bed (on my left side) and see what happened. Once on the bed, I asked if our midwife could see anything and she said she saw "bulging."

Once I was on the bed, all I felt like doing was pushing. I didn't think I was pushing the baby out; it's just how I felt during a contraction. I couldn't stop myself or my body, really. After a contraction ended, I kept on pushing. Our midwife suggested I rest until the next one so I would have energy.

During a contraction, she suggested I hold on to one leg so that I felt like I had control or someplace to put my hand. So during a contraction I would push, not really thinking that this was the actual pushing that brings the baby, but rather just what my body was wanting to do, perhaps for relief from the contraction.

I still felt clueless to the fact that the baby was coming soon. I would rest between contractions. At the start of a new one, I would say "help" because I felt like I couldn't lift my leg up to get a hold on it. I remember kind of letting some loud sounds out and apologizing for it. Our midwife said "you make whatever noises you need to make."

During one contraction my water broke; it was 11:53 p.m. It was clear fluid so all was good. I kept pushing and then relaxing and at one point I asked our midwife how dilated I was and she said something like "you are 10, you are there, you are doing it." It still hadn't dawned on me that I was that far along and ready to be pushing my baby out, which is what I was doing anyway.

Another time during this pushing phase I asked what position the baby was in, since she had been posterior during my entire pregnancy and it was a concern of mine. Our midwife answered with something like, "This baby is coming out."

Shortly after my water broke I could literally feel the baby slide down a long way, which was an odd feeling and I remember saying something like "oh my." Then they said the head was starting to show and asked if I wanted to touch her head. When I felt it I think I said "Oh my gosh" because it wasn't just the top of the head I felt but some of the sides as well. Again, I had no idea she was almost out of me!

I remember our midwife saying at some point "In the next few minutes (or next few pushes, I can't remember) you will have your baby in your arms." And I said "Really?" I was stunned. Again, I just didn't comprehend that she was almost here!

I remember someone saying "the head is out" and then not long after that my baby was being placed on my chest! It was the most amazing feeling! I still couldn't believe she was here already! Born exactly 10 minutes after my water broke, at 12:03 a.m! And she felt so tiny on my chest. I thought she was going to be a tiny baby, but she ended up weighing 8 lbs. I was giddy with emotion and was laughing some weird kind of high-pitched laugh that everyone asked if I was laughing or crying!

We woke Griffin up about an hour after she was born and he was instantly in love with her. It was so cute to see! I am still in shock about how quick of a birth it ended up being (not counting the day+ of early labor). Two hours after we called the midwife our baby was born!

Our midwife said later that her head was showing quite a bit in the posterior position when she saw it rotate 180 degrees and she was born anterior.

Even though I didn't feel as calm and focused as I did during our son's birth, I was so happy with our home birth! It was awesome to be able to stay in our comfortable home and it was a great place to recover after the birth. Once everyone left (about 2:40 a.m.) all four of us cuddled up in our bed and fell asleep. I was the last one to fall asleep; I guess there was still so much adrenaline running through me.

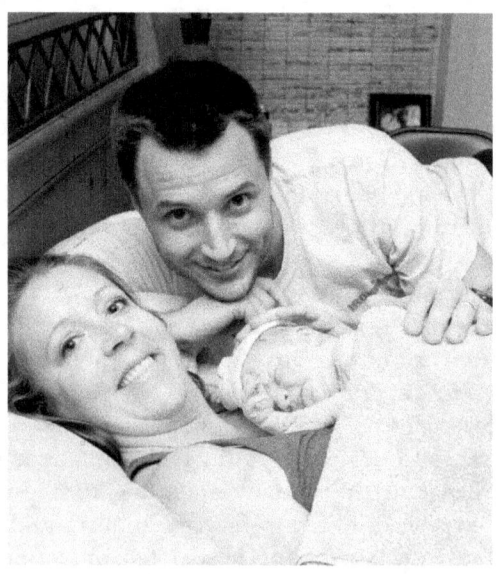

START NOW TO CULTIVATE YOUR COURAGE FOR THE NATURAL BIRTH OF YOUR DREAMS

To have a natural birth remember: control what you can and let the rest go. Start now by taking action on the things you can control:

** **Your determination.** Why do you want to have a natural childbirth? Do some soul searching to discover and ignite your determination.

** **Your knowledge about natural birth.** Start reading! Buy one or two of the highly recommended books (or check them out from a library). Also, find a natural childbirth class and sign up.

** **Your caregiver and birth location.** Gather questions and start interviewing potential caregivers to find one that will best support you. If you have a caregiver, start talking about natural birth.

** **Your support.** Go to the Natural Unmedicated Childbirth forum at Babycenter.com, sign up, introduce yourself, and join in the conversations. (community.babycenter.com/groups/a424255/natural_unmedicated_childbirth)

** **Your mind.** Find positive affirmations for a safe, healthy pregnancy and birth, make a list, and start reading it daily. Make a list of any fears or concerns you have and find someone to talk to about them.

** **Your breathing.** Practice meditation or yoga to learn breathing and relaxation techniques. Some natural childbirth classes also focus on the importance of learning breathing and relaxation techniques for labor.

** **Your diet and exercise.** Start keeping a food journal; after a few weeks share it with your caregiver. Learn and discuss ways to implement an optimal healthy pregnancy diet. Also discuss an appropriate exercise plan.

** **Bonus Materials:** Download my free gifts to you!

ADVICE FROM NATURAL BIRTHING MOMS

I received so much great advice from many natural birthing moms that I wanted to share even more of it with you. Notice how the advice involves all five keys to having a natural birth.

Determination – Information – Support – Belief – Prepare

"Be determined! Believe in yourself and your body. Also make sure that your husband and your providers are on the same page—extremely important!" – Erin

"Be determined, research and know your stuff, be confident because it's not the norm and you may have to 'fight' to be successful. Have a supportive team." – Arusi

"Educate yourself. Believe in yourself. Find a support system. Be kind to yourself." – Kelly

"Do your research, and know your options." – Alicia

"Take time to get to know the birthing process and have your partner do the same so they can best support you. And remember that you deserve informed consent." – Sandra

"Read up on it. Get knowledgeable. Talk to a midwife and ask a lot of questions." – Holly

"Education, choose a care provider that practices evidence-based care and uses shared decision-making processes, process your fears, be flexible but have positive expectations." – Stacy

"Own your own choices, and chose a birthplace and support people who will help you to do things the way you want." – Jamie

"Make sure you hire birth professionals that will support your plan for a natural birth." – Dianthe

"Hire a doula if you are birthing in a hospital, attend birth classes that encourage and focus on natural birth." – Jennifer

"DO NOT let other people bring you down my telling you that you cannot achieve it. Surround yourself with people that support your choice." – Julia

"Believe in yourself. Believe in your body. Believe this is what women were made to do. Read Ina May's Guide to Childbirth. Take control of your environment and don't be afraid to demand exactly what you want." – April

"Your body was made for this and every contraction gets you closer to holding your baby." – Stephanie

"Trust yourself. You can do it. It will be the most amazing thing you've ever done." – Anonymous

"Believe you can do it and don't listen to skeptics or nay-sayers. You are stronger than you think!" – Malisa

"Believe in yourself, believe in your baby, and follow your heart always." – Kali

"Your body is capable of it! Just believe in yourself and in your body. You can

do it!" – Abbey

"Women are strong; we can do this and have done this since the beginning of time." – Karen P.

"Just prepare your body and mind for it by exercising, meditating, and eating right." – Amber

"Practice breathing! If nothing else, practice your breathing techniques to help you cope, and surround yourself with a team of people who can support your decisions." – Tabitha

"Get a doula, prepare yourself, stay active, find a midwife/physician who is supportive, and stick to your guns; you can do it." – Katie

"Get a doula, take good, non-hospital based childbirth classes, envision the birth you want, and make a detailed birth plan to that effect." – Delayna

"Wait as long as possible before going to the hospital, hire a doula (!!!!!), and drink lots of red raspberry leaf tea." – Lauren

"Prepare, have a birth plan." – Cathryn

"Don't just expect it to happen. It's extremely difficult and requires some mental preparation so that you don't freak out the moment once the real contractions start." – Jenny

"Envision your healthy and alert baby coming into the world on their own terms and what a wonderful beginning this will be for your relationship. It's so worth it." – Angela

QUICK REFERENCE TIPS FOR NATURAL BIRTH IN A HOSPITAL

"Birth should not be a time in a woman's life when she has to FIGHT for anything." – Carla Hartley

Since I did not birth my babies in a hospital, these tips come from my friends who have had natural births in hospitals as well as from 11+ years of researching birth on my own.

** Let labor start on its own.

** Labor at home as long as you can.

** Bring your **confidence in your ability** to have a natural birth, and share this confidence with staff.

** Share what this natural birth means to you with your nurses, and **ask their help** in being your advocate.

** **Understand your options** ahead of time. You will be more prepared to assert your wishes if you know what obstacles may be ahead.

** Make a plan for support. Make sure your partner knows how to support you and is comfortable advocating for you with the staff. Consider hiring a doula.

** Make a plan for **privacy and comfort**. Turn your phone off. Wear your own clothes. Keep lights and voices low (bring a night light). Bring your own blanket for the bed. Use an aromatherapy spray with a pleasing scent. Have special music playing. When hospital staff walk into the room, they will automatically know that something different and special is happening.

** Hang a **sign on the door** of your room letting staff know that a natural birth is in progress. Each time they enter the room, they will be reminded. (Print a couple, in case it disappears.) Good news! I made you one you can print yourself; check out the next page.

** Learn breathing and relaxation techniques. **Deep breathing and a calm mind** cannot be taken away from you.

** When speaking to hospital staff, **assert what you want** instead of being accusatory or debating statistics. Always speak directly, with respect and courtesy (and confidence).

** Remember: **You have a choice and a voice.**

I CAN AND I WILL

THANK YOU! (AND FREE GIFTS)

Thank you for purchasing my book. I know you have many books to choose from on natural birth, but you took a chance with mine. It's my most sincere hope that it has helped you (and will continue to help you) on your journey to a natural childbirth.

If you liked what you read, I would love your help. Please take a moment to write a review for this book on Amazon. (AwakeningWillow.com/ICanIWillAmazonReview)

Free Gifts

As a thank you for your purchase of this book, I am offering several free gifts to help you achieve your natural birth, including:

** Birthing Room Door Sign: Let anyone entering your room know that a natural birth is in progress. This sign was designed by me and is printable by you. (PDF)

** Labor Support Sheet: Many reminders and reassurances for your partner to help you during labor on one page. (PDF)

To receive your free gifts, head over to AwakeningWillow.com/ICanIWillBookGifts.

Reminder

Regardless of whether you have a natural birth or not, I hope you find benefit in the process of self-discovery and personal growth that is inherent in planning a natural birth.

You have changed through the effort you expended in going out of your comfort zone, asserting your views when they may not be the norm, learning new things about birth and your body. Questioning, stretching, growing.

And now be ready to change even more once you become a mother. Motherhood is like birth; not easy, but worth it. It's all beautiful and it's all worth it.

Everything is hard before it's easy.

Best wishes for a beautiful birth,
Wendy

AwakeningWillow.com

"When you are inspired by some great purpose, some extraordinary project, all your thoughts break their bonds: Your mind transcends limitations, your consciousness expands in every direction, and you find yourself in a new, great, and wonderful world. Dormant forces, faculties and talents become alive, and you discover yourself to be a greater person by far than you ever dreamed yourself to be." – Patañjali

ACKNOWLEDGEMENTS

There are times in our lives when we need support and encouragement and times when we can offer support and encouragement to others. The writing of this book has granted me both opportunities, and for that I am grateful.

You are reading this book because you want support and encouragement in your desire to have a natural birth; and I am happy to offer that to you. Hopefully my support has helped you find your *courage and strength* to keep going.

I asked for help during the writing process and was humbled by the support and encouragement I received. Every time a request was met with a "yes," I was not only surprised and grateful but filled with *courage and strength* to keep going.

My deepest gratitude goes to my husband, David, for holding space for me as I quit writing this book 100 times. His support and encouragement helped me start writing this book 101 times.

Thank you to my friends for sharing their natural birthing stories, reviewing my book, and offering encouragement. Juliana, Carey Sue, Amy, Andrea, Stacy, Kat, D'Lynn: your support and encouragement meant the world to me. Thank you to my friend Katie: your awesome editing skills, suggestions, and encouragement helped me through the vulnerable final stages of the creative process. Sisterhood is powerful; thanks for being part of mine.

A very sincere thank you goes to the women who answered my survey questions and allowed me to share their stories. Their "yeses" not only helped my book be more able to help others, but has changed us from strangers to friends in my heart. Thank you Abbey, Adriana, Alex, Alicia, Amber, Angela, Annette, April, Arusi, Ashley, Bonnie, Bryn, Cathryn, Chenae, Christina, Courtney, Dana, Delayna, Delilah, Dianthe, Elanna, Emily, Erin, Fonda, Grace, Holly, Jamie, Jen, Jennifer, Jenny, Jessica, Julia, Kali, Karen H., Karen P., Kate, Katie, Kayla, Kelly, Kimberly, Kristen, Laurel, Lauren, Leah, Malisa, Margaret, Marissa, Melanie, Michelle, Mirja, Monique, Nadine, Nina, Rachel, Rosa, Samantha, Sandra, Sara, Stephanie, Susan, Tabitha, Talitha, Tatiana, and a few others who wish to remain anonymous. Your gift to me is now a gift to many other women as well.

I'm even grateful for those who were not supportive. Each odd comment I received led to deeper reflection on my intention, approach, and content, ultimately leading to a better book.

Asking for support is a practice in vulnerability. Offering support keeps up each other's courage. By sharing your time, thoughts, and opinions you kept up my courage.

What we help each other achieve, we share.

Together. That's a good place to be.

RECOMMENDED RESOURCES: BOOKS, WEBSITES, ARTICLES

More Books

** **Active Birth**, by Janet Balaskas

** **The Birth Book: Everything You Need to Know to Have a Safe and Satisfying Birth**, by William Sears and Martha Sears

** **Birthing From Within: An Extra-Ordinary Guide to Childbirth Preparation**, by Pam England and Rob Horowitz

** **The Birth Partner**, by Penny Simkin

** **Childbirth Without Fear**, by Grantly Dick-Read

** **The Doula Book**, by Marshall Klaus, John Kennell, and Phyllis Klaus

** **Easing Labor Pain**, by Adrienne Lieberman

** **Gentle Birth Choices**, by Barbara Harper

** **Gentle Birth, Gentle Mothering: A Doctor's Guide to Natural Childbirth and Gentle Early Parenting Choices**, by Sarah J. Buckley, MD

** **A Good Birth, A Safe Birth: Choosing and Having the Childbirth Experience You Want**, by Diana Korte and Roberta Scaer

** **Husband-Coached Childbirth: The Bradley Method of Natural Childbirth**, by Robert Bradley

** **Journey Into Motherhood: Inspirational Stories of Natural Birth**, by Sheri L. Menelli

** **Mindful Birthing: Training the Mind, Body, and Heart for Childbirth and Beyond**, by Nancy Bardacke

** **Mothering the Mother: How a Doula Can Help You Have a Shorter, Easier, and Healthier Birth**, by Marshall Klaus, John Kennell, and Phyllis Klaus

** **The Nurturing Touch at Birth**, by Paulina Perez

** **Pushed: The Painful Truth About Childbirth and Modern Maternity Care**, by Jennifer Block

** **Your Best Birth: Know All Your Options, Discover the Natural Choices, and Take Back the Birth Experience**, by Ricki Lake and Abby Epstein.

Websites

BirthCenters.org
BirthingNaturally.net

Cfmidwifery.org
ChildbirthConnection.org
ChoicesinChildbirth.org
EvidenceBasedBirth.com
GivingBirthWithConfidence.org
HumanRightsinChildbirth.com
ImprovingBirth.org
MotherFriendly.org (Coalition for Improving Maternity Services)
MothersNaturally.org
ScienceAndSensibility.org
SpinningBabies.com
TrustBirth.com

Articles

The most scientific birth is often the least technological one.

theatlantic.com/health/archive/2012/03/the-most-scientific-birth-is-often-the-least-technological-birth/254420

Epidural Epidemic

mothering.com/articles/epidural-epidemic

How painful is childbirth?

birthingnaturally.net/birth/pain/how.html

How to Help a Woman in Labor

thejoyofthis.com/2011/12/07/how-to-help-a-woman-in-labor

Preparing for Natural Hospital Birth

mamabirth.com/2012/01/preparing-for-natural-hospital-birth.html

Hormonal Physiology of Childbearing: Evidence and Implications for Women, Babies, and Maternity Care

transform.childbirthconnection.org/reports/physiology

Safe, Healthy Birth: What Every Pregnant Woman Needs Know

ncbi.nlm.nih.gov/pmc/articles/PMC2730905

Evidence-Based Maternity Care: What It Is and What It Can Achieve

childbirthconnection.com/pdfs/evidence-based-maternity-care.pdf

How to Stay Healthy and Low Risk During Pregnancy and Birth

midwiferytoday.com/articles/stayhealthy.asp

Nutrition During Pregnancy

midwiferytoday.com/articles/nutritionpreg.asp

Preventing Complications with Nutrition

midwiferytoday.com/articles/nutrition.asp

Advancing Normal Birth

motherfriendly.org/resources/documents/cims_evidence_basis.pdf

"No Thank You" – A Guide to Informed Decision Making

42weeks.ie/2013/08/07/no-thank-you-a-guide-to-informed-decison-making

I CAN AND I WILL

CHAPTER NOTES

Introduction

1. Seth Godin quote.

Godin, Seth. *What to do When It's Your Turn (and it's always your turn)*. The Domino Project, 2014. Print.

2. Women who are more confident in their ability to cope with labor experience less pain during labor.

Lowe NK. "The nature of labor pain." *American Journal of Obstetrics and Gynecology* 186.5 (2002):S16-24.

Chapter 1: From Desire to Determination

1. Birth numbers for hospital, home, and birth center births.

Martin, Joyce, Brady Hamilton, Michelle Osterman, Sally Curtin, and TJ Mathews. *Births: Final data for 2013*. National Vital Statistics Reports. Volume 64 Number 1. Hyattsville, MD: National Center for Health Statistics. 2015. CDC. Web. 4 July 2015.

2. In one survey, 17% of women who birthed at hospitals reported using no pain medication during labor.

Declercq ER, Sakala C, Corry MP, Applebaum S, Herrlich A. *Listening to Mothers[SM] III: Pregnancy and Birth*. New York: Childbirth Connection, May 2013.

Chapter 2: Be Informed, Be Inspired

1. According to one study, women who were least afraid of childbirth and viewed it as a natural process had the highest rate of unassisted vaginal births.

Haines, Helen M., Christine Rubertsson, Julie F. Pallant, and Ingegerd Hildingsson. "The Influence of Women's Fear, Attitudes and Beliefs of Childbirth on Mode and Experience of Birth." *BMC Pregnancy and Childbirth* 12.55 (2012): n. pag. BioMedCentral. Web. 4 July 2015.

2. While beneficial when complications arise, many common medical interventions are used when they are not truly needed. Unnecessary medical interventions used during labor and childbirth can have unintended effects

because they interfere with the normal physiology of labor and birth.

Lothian, Juduth A., Debby Amis, and Jeannette Crenshaw. "Care Practice #4: No Routine Interventions." *Journal of Perinatal Education* 16.3 (2007): 29-34. PMC Web. 09 May 2015.

"Cascade of Intervention in Childbirth." *Childbirth Connection.* National Partnership for Women & Families. N.p., 11 April 2011. Web. 09 May 2015.

Induction:

3. Synthetic oxytocin can interfere with the mother's natural hormones during labor, causing contractions that are longer, stronger, and closer together. This can be harder on the baby than natural contractions.

Goer, Henci. *The Thinking Woman's Guide to a Better Birth.* New York: Berkley, 1999. Print.

4. Induction of labor usually involves an IV line, continuous electronic fetal monitoring (EFM), restriction of movement, and restriction of eating and drinking. Women are more likely to request an epidural during induced labors.

King, Valerie J., Rachel Pilliod, and Alison Little. *Rapid Review: Elective Induction of Labor.* Portland: Center for Evidence-based Policy, 2010. http://www.ohsu.edu/xd/research/centers-institutes/evidence-based-policy-center/med/index.cfm. Web.

5. Some inductions are medically necessary but many inductions are due to reasons of convenience or other non-medical rationale, such as the baby is full term, wanting to be done with the pregnancy, or wanting to control timing.

Declercq ER, Sakala C, Corry MP, Applebaum S, Herrlich A. *Listening to Mothers* III: Pregnancy and Birth. New York: Childbirth Connection, May 2013.

6. Be aware that some providers use misoprostol (Cytotec) for induction and cervical ripening even though it has not been approved by the FDA for this purpose. Once started, its effects cannot be stopped. It can have serious side effects, such as uterine hyperstimulation.

Hofmeyr GJ, Gülmezoglu AM, Pileggi C. "Vaginal misoprostol for cervical ripening and induction of labour." *Cochrane Database Systemic Reviews.* Issue10 (2010) Art. No. CD000941. DOI:

10.1002/14651858.CD000941.pub2.

Goer, Henci. *The Thinking Woman's Guide to a Better Birth*. New York: Berkley, 1999. Print.

7. Sometimes a provider's concern about the size of the baby leads mothers to choose induction, a practice that is not supported by best evidence.

Mozurkewich E, Chilimigras J, Koepke E, Keeton K, King VJ. "Indications for induction of labour: A best-evidence review." *BJOG*. 116.5 (2009):626-636. PMC. Web. 4 July 2015.

8. Eating dates during the last month of pregnancy may help reduce the need for induction or augmentation of labor.

Al-Kuran O, Al-Mehaisen L, Bawadi H, Beitawi S, Amarin Z. "The effect of late pregnancy consumption of date fruit on labour and delivery." *Journal of Obstetrics and Gynaecology*. 31.1 (2011):29-31. doi: 10.3109/01443615.2010.522267.

Artificial Rupture of Membranes:

9. Due to an increased risk of infection from repeated vaginal exams, once your bag of water is broken your care provider will probably want your baby to be born within a certain amount of time (usually 12-24 hours). This can increase the use of other interventions such as Pitocin, EFM, IV, restriction of movement, and may possibly lead to a cesarean.

Goer, Henci. *The Thinking Woman's Guide to a Better Birth*. New York: Berkley, 1999. Print.

Johnson N et al. "Randomised trial comparing a policy of early with selective amniotomy in uncomplicated labour at term." *British Journal of Obstetrics Gynaecology* 104.3 (1997):340-346.

Routine Continuous Electronic Fetal Monitoring:

10. Compared with intermittent auscultation, routine continuous EFM increases the risk of cesarean for mothers while having no significant improvement in the overall perinatal death rate.

Alfirevic Z, Devane D, Gyte GM. "Continuous cardiotocography (CTG) as a form of electronic fetal monitoring (EFM) for fetal assessment during labour." *Cochrane Database Systemic Reviews*. Issue 5 (2013) Art. No. CD006066. doi: 10.1002/14651858.CD006066.pub2

11. The American Congress of Obstetricians and Gynecologists (ACOG)

says either intermittent listening with a stethoscope or continuous EFM may be used for women who don't have complications.

ACOG. "ACOG Practice Bulletin 106: Intrapartum fetal heart rate monitoring: nomenclature, interpretation, and general management principles." *Obstetrics and Gynecology*. 114.1 (2009):192-202. doi: 10.1097/AOG.0b013e3181aef106.
https://docs.google.com/file/d/0B1t0K9SZCmm0T051S3FrTlpYMzg/edit

Routine Intravenous (IV) Fluids:

12. Routine IV use restricts movement, may lead to fluid overload (which can lead to problems with breastfeeding, baby losing weight, baby with jaundice, fluid in mom's and/or baby's lungs), and may contribute to low blood sugar in newborns.

Goer, Henci. *The Thinking Woman's Guide to a Better Birth*. New York: Berkley, 1999. Print.

13. The American Society of Anesthesiologists (ASA) and the ACOG recommend allowing low-risk laboring women to drink clear liquids.

American Society of Anesthesiologists Task Force on Obstetric Anesthesia. "Practice guidelines for obstetric anesthesia: An updated report by the American Society of Anesthesiologists Task Force on Obstetric Anesthesia." *Anesthesiology*. 106.4 (2007):843–863.

ACOG "ACOG Practice Bulletin 36: Obstetric analgesia and anesthesia." *Obstetrics and Gynecology*. 100.1 (2002):177–191. http://www.ncbi.nlm.nih.gov/pubmed/12100826

Lothian, Juduth A., Debby Amis, and Jeannette Crenshaw. "Care Practice #4: No Routine Interventions." *Journal of Perinatal Education* 16.3 (2007): 29-34. PMC. Web. 09 May 2015.

Epidural:

14. Epidurals interfere with birth hormones, slowing labor and making pushing more difficult; all of which can lead to increased use of vaginal instruments (forceps or vacuum-extraction), episiotomy, and a cesarean. Epidural drugs do reach the baby and can cause disturbances of the fetal heart rate and other adverse effects.

Buckley, Sarah J. "Ecstatic Birth: The Hormonal Blueprint of Labor," *Mothering* March/April 2002 http://www.mothering.com/articles/ecstatic-birth/ Web. 25 May 2015.

Buckley, Sarah J. *Hormonal Physiology of Childbearing: Evidence and Implications for Women, Babies, and Maternity Care.* Washington, D.C.: Childbirth Connection Programs, National Partnership for Women & Families, January 2015. http://childbirthconnection.org/HormonalPhysiology

Goer, Henci. *The Thinking Woman's Guide to a Better Birth.* New York: Berkley, 1999. Print.

15. Initiation of breastfeeding can be more difficult after epidural use.

Goer, Henci. *The Thinking Woman's Guide to a Better Birth.* New York: Berkley, 1999. Print.

Riordan, J., Gross, A., Angeron, J., Krumwiede, B., Melin, J. "Effect of Labor Pain Relief Medication on Neonatal Suckling and Breastfeeding Duration," *Journal of Human Lactation* 16.1 (2000): 7-12.

Ransjo-Arvidson A.B., Matthiesen, A.S., Lilja, G., Missen, E., Widstrom, A.M., Uvnas-Moberg, K., "Maternal Analgesia during Labor Disturbs Newborn Behavior: Effects on Breastfeeding, Temperature, and Crying," *Birth* 28.1 (2001): 20-21. PMC. Web. 4 July 2015.

Restriction of Movement:

16. Movement such as walking and changing positions can relieve pain and shorten labor.

Lothian, Juduth A., Debby Amis, and Jeannette Crenshaw. "Care Practice #4: No Routine Interventions." *Journal of Perinatal Education* 16.3 (2007): 29-34. PMC. Web. 09 May 2015.

17. Walking in early labor can reduce the chances of a cesarean.

Storton, Sharon. "Step 4: Provides the Birthing Woman With Freedom of Movement to Walk, Move, Assume Positions of Her Choice: The Coalition for Improving Maternity Services:" *The Journal of Perinatal Education* 16.1 (2007): 25S–27S. PMC. Web. 25 May 2015.

Chapter 3: Find Your Support and Your Strength Will Follow

1. The majority of pregnancies (70-80%) are considered low-risk.

World Health Organization *Care in normal birth: Report of a technical work group.* Geneva: World Health Organization, 1996. WHO. Web. 4 July 2015.

2. Options for Caregivers: Midwives

"Choosing a Caregiver, Options: Midwives for Maternity Care." *Childbirth Connection*. National Partnership for Women & Families. N.p., 17 January 2008. Web. 24 July 2015.

3. Options for Caregivers: Physicians

"Choosing a Caregiver, Options: Family Physicians and Obstetricians for Maternity Care." *Childbirth Connection*. National Partnership for Women & Families. N.p., 3 March 2011. Web. 24 July 2015.

4. Having continuous support during labor and birth has many benefits, especially when the provider is not part of the hospital staff or the woman's social network such as with a doula. In addition to having slightly shorter labors, women with continuous support during labor were:
     ** less likely to use any pain medication
     ** less likely to have a cesarean section
     ** more likely to have spontaneous vaginal birth (no cesarean, vacuum-extraction, or forceps)
     ** less likely to rate their childbirth experience negatively

Hodnett ED, Gates S, Hofmeyr GJ, Sakala C. "Continuous support for women during childbirth." *Cochrane Database of Systemic Reviews*. Issue 10 (2012) Art. No. CD003766. DOI: 10.1002/14651858.CD003766.pub4.

Chapter 4: Nurture a Belief in Yourself

1. Some common fears may include fear of pain, fear of losing control, fear of problems with the baby, and fear of your wishes not being respected, among others.

McGrath, Kathryn. "Continuing Education Module The Courage to Birth." *The Journal of Perinatal Education* 21.2 (2012): 72–79. PMC. Web. 23 June 2015.

2. Hypnobabies affirmations.

Tuschhoff, Kerry. "Joyful Pregnancy Affirmations." *Hypnobabies*. Hypnobabies Home-Study Course, n.d. CD.

Chapter 5: Plan and Prepare: A Great Paradox of Birth

1. Hopefully your caregiver is providing nutritional education and counseling at your prenatal appointments, as this has been shown to have health benefits for the mother as well as the baby. Benefits of excellent prenatal nutrition: (list)

Girard AW, Olude O. "Nutrition education and counselling provided during pregnancy: effects on maternal, neonatal and child health outcomes." *Paediatric and Perinatal Epidemiology*. 26.s1 (2012):191-204. PubMed. Web. 24 June 2015

Englund-Ögge, Linda et al. "Maternal Dietary Patterns and Preterm Delivery: Results from Large Prospective Cohort Study." *BMJ: British Medical Journal* 348 (2014): g1446. PMC. Web. 4 July 2015.

Brewer, Tom. *Metabolic Toxemia of Late Pregnancy*. New Canaan, Connecticut: Keats Publishing Inc., 1982. Print.

Lechtig A, Yarrough C, Delgado H, Martorell R, Klein RE, Béhar M. "Effect of moderate maternal malnutrition on the placenta." *American Journal of Obstetrics and Gynecology* 123.2 (1975):191-201. PMC. Web. 25 June 2015.

Nagata C, Nakamura K, Wada K, Oba S, Hayashi M, Takeda N, Yasuda K. "Association of dietary fat, vegetables and antioxidant micronutrients with skin ageing in Japanese women" *British Journal of Nutrition* 103.10 (2010):1493-1498. Web. 25 June 2015.

Segger D, Matthies A, Saldeen T. "Supplementation with Eskimo Skin Care improves skin elasticity in women. A pilot study." *The Journal of Dermatological Treatment* 19.5 (2008):279-283. PMC. Web. 25 June 2015.

2. The basics include eating high-quality foods from all the food groups, with enough protein, healthy fats, adequate salt (to taste), and filtered water (to thirst)—while reducing empty calorie junk foods.

Haas, Amy V. "Nutrition During Pregnancy" *Having a Baby Today*. Spring 2002. *Midwifery Today*. Web. 26 June 2015.

3. Women who exercise during pregnancy handle the work of labor easier, tend to have shorter labors, have an easier time pushing baby out, need fewer medical interventions, and physically recover easier.

Perales M, Calabria I, Lopez C, Franco E, Coteron J, Barakat R. "Regular Exercise Throughout Pregnancy Is Associated With a Shorter First Stage of Labor." *American Journal of Health Promotion*. 2015 Jan 23. [Epub ahead of print]. PMC. Web. 26 June 2015.

Rice PL, Fort IL. "The relationship of maternal exercise on labor, delivery and health of the newborn." *Journal of Sports Medicine and Physical Fitness*.

31.1 (1991):95–99. PMC. Web. 26 June 2015.

Clapp, James F. *Exercising Through Your Pregnancy*. Champaign: Human Kinetics, 1998. Print.

Sternfeld B, Quesenberry J, Eskenazi B, Newman L. "Exercise during pregnancy and pregnancy outcome." *Medicine and Science in Sports and Exercise*. 27.5 (1995):634–640. PMC. Web. 26 June 2015.

May, Linda E. *Physiology of Prenatal Exercise and Fetal Development*. New York: Springer-Verlag, 2012. DOI: 10.1007/978-1-4614-3408-5_2.

Hammer R, Perkins J, Parr R. "Exercise During the Childbearing Year." *The Journal of Perinatal Education*. 9.1 (2000): 1-14. PMC. Web. 26 June 2015.

4. Doing Kegel exercises during pregnancy has been associated with easier labors.

Salvesen K. "Randomised controlled trial of pelvic floor muscle training during pregnancy" *British Medical Journal*. 329.7462 (2004):378-380. PMC. Web. 26 June 2015.

5. Most posterior babies rotate in labor.

Gardberg M, Laakkonen E, Salevaara M. "Intrapartum sonography and persistent occiput posterior position: a study of 408 deliveries." *Obstetrics and Gynecology*. 91.5 Pt1 (1998):746-749. PMC. Web. 26 June 2015.

6. Moxibustion has been also used successfully to turn breech babies.

Cardini F., Weixin H. "Moxibustion for correction of breech presentation: A randomized controlled trial." *Journal of the American Medical Association* 280.18 (1998):1580-1584. PMC. Web. 26 June 2015.

Coyle ME, Smith CA, Peat B. "Cephalic version by moxibustion for breech presentation." *Cochrane Database of Systematic Reviews* Issue 5 (2012) Art. No. CD003928. DOI: 10.1002/14651858.CD003928.pub3.

7. The chiropractic Webster technique has also been used successfully to turn breech babies.

Kunau, PL. "Application of the Webster In-Utero Constraint Technique: A Case Series" *Journal of Clinical Chiropractic Pediatrics* 3.1 (1998). Icpa4kids.org. Web. 26 June 2015.

Pistolese RA. "The Webster Technique: a chiropractic technique with obstetric implications." *Journal of Manipulative Physiological Therapeutics.* 25.6 (2002): E1-9. PubMed. Web. 26 June 2015.

8. Routine chiropractic care can be helpful for comfort during pregnancy, but it can also reduce labor time.

Borggren CL. "Pregnancy and chiropractic: a narrative review of the literature." *Journal of Chiropractic Medicine* 6.2 (2007):70-74. PMC. Web. 26 June 2015.

9. Some studies have shown that performing a perineal massage in the last few weeks of pregnancy can help prevent tearing during birth, especially for first-time moms.

Shipman MK, Boniface DR, Tefft ME, McCloghry F. "Antenatal perineal massage and subsequent perineal outcomes: A randomized trial." *British Journal of Obstetrics and Gynaecology* 104.7 (1997):787-791. PMC. Web. 28 June 2015.

Labrecque M, Eason E, Marcoux S, Lemieux F, Pinault JJ, Feldman P, Laperrière L. "Randomized controlled trial of prevention of perineal trauma by perineal massage during pregnancy." *American Journal of Obstetrics and Gynecology* 180.3 (1999):593-600. PMC. Web. 28 June 2015.

10. Regular exercise is effective in preparing and strengthening the perineal area.

Gordon H, Logue M. "Perineal muscle function after childbirth." *Lancet* 2.8447 (1985):123-125. PMC. Web. 28 June 2015.

11. The side-lying (lateral) position has been shown to be the birth position with the highest rate of intact perineum.

Shorten A, Donsante J, Shorten B. "Birth position, accoucheur, and perineal outcomes: informing women about choices for vaginal birth." *Birth* 29.1 (2002):18-27. PMC. Web. 28 June 2015.

Uterus Toning and Cervical Ripening

12. There are several traditional herbal supplements that are favorites in the midwifery world for toning the uterus.

McFarlin BL, Gibson MH, O'Rear J, Harman P. "A national survey of herbal preparation use by nurse-midwives for labor stimulation: Review of the literature and recommendations for practice." *Journal of Nurse-*

Midwifery 44.3 (1999):205-216. PMC. Web. 28 June 2015.

13. Drinking red raspberry leaf tea in late pregnancy is believed to tone the uterus and help make the contractions more effective during labor.

Parsons M, Simpson , Ponton T. "Raspberry leaf and its effect on labour: safety and efficacy." *Australian College of Midwives Incorporated Journal.* 12.3 (1999):20-25. PuMC. Web. 28 June 2015.

Simpson M, Parsons M, Greenwood J, Wade K. "Raspberry leaf in pregnancy: its safety and efficacy in labor." *Journal of Midwifery and Women's Health.* 46.2 (2001):51-59. PuMC. Web. 28 June 2015.

14. Taking EPO capsules late in pregnancy is believed to help ripen the cervix, due to the actions of the prostaglandins produced.

McFarlin BL, Gibson MH, O'Rear J, Harman P. "A national survey of herbal preparation use by nurse-midwives for labor stimulation: Review of the literature and recommendations for practice." *Journal of Nurse-Midwifery* 44.3 (1999):205-216. PMC. Web. 28 June 2015.

15. Eating dates during the last month of pregnancy may help shorten labor as well as reduce the need for induction or augmentation of labor.

Al-Kuran O, Al-Mehaisen L, Bawadi H, Beitawi S, Amarin Z. "The effect of late pregnancy consumption of date fruit on labour and delivery." *Journal of Obstetrics and Gynaecology.* 31.1 (2011):29-31. PMC. Web. 28 June 2015.

Chapter 6: Labor at Home as Long as Possible

1. Most labors do not start with your water breaking (only about 8% do).

Marowitz A, Jordan R. "Midwifery management of prelabor rupture of membranes at term." *Journal of Midwifery and Women's Health.* 52.3 (2007):199-206. PMC. Web. 28 June 2015.

2. Labors can last an average of 16 hours for first time moms.

Smith, Kira. "Every Labor is Different" *Pregnancy and Baby.* n.d.:n. Pag. Web. 28 June 2015.

Chapter 7: Turn Fear Into Acceptance

1. The uterus has two opposing muscle layers that work together during labor.

Griffin, Nancy. "The Epidural Express: Real Reasons Not to Jump

Aboard." *Mothering* Spring 1997: 46-55.

2. Famous midwife Ina May Gaskin notes a connection between tension in the mouth and jaw and tension in the cervix.

Gaskin, Ina May. *Ina May's Guide to Childbirth*. New York: Bantam Dell, 2003. Print.

Chapter 8: Stay Hydrated and Nourished

1. Studies show there is no evidence of harm from eating and drinking during labor.

Singata M, Tranmer J, Gyte GML. "Restricting oral fluid and food intake during labour." *Cochrane Database of Systemic Reviews*. Issue 8 (2013). Art. No. CD003930. DOI: 10.1002/14651858.CD003930.pub3.

Chapter 9: Comfort and Coping Techniques

1. The **more confident** you are that you will be able to cope, the **less pain** you will feel.

Lowe NK. "Maternal confidence in coping with labor: A self-efficacy concept." *Journal of Obstetric, Gynecologic, and Neonatal Nursing* 20.6 (1991):457-463. PMC. Web. 2 July 2015.

Chapter 10: Birth in a Position You Choose

1. Evidence supports the use of upright and side-lying positions as safer and healthier for mom and baby, with results of shorter pushing time, fewer forceps or vacuum births, fewer episiotomies, less severe pain, and fewer abnormal fetal heart rate patterns.

Lothian, Judith A. "Safe, Healthy Birth: What Every Pregnant Woman Needs to Know." *The Journal of Perinatal Education* 18.3 (2009): 48–54. PMC. Web. 3 July 2015.

Gupta JK, Hofmeyr GJ, Shehmar M. "Position in the second stage of labour for women without epidural anaesthesia." *Cochrane Database of Systematic Reviews* Issue 5. (2012) Art. No. CD002006. DOI: 10.1002/14651858.CD002006.pub3.

2. The supine/lithotomy (flat-on-back) position is the most commonly used position in vaginal births in hospitals (68%); a close second is the reclining (or semi-sitting) position (23%).

Declercq ER, Sakala C, Corry MP, Applebaum S, Herrlich A. *Listening to Mothers^SM III: Pregnancy and Birth*. New York: Childbirth Connection,

May 2013.

3. [The supine/lithotomy positions] are used mostly for the convenience of the hospital staff.

Oxorn, Harry *Human Labor and Birth* Ontario: McGraw-Hill, 1986.

3. There are several disadvantages of birthing on your back:
    ** more painful than other positions:

De Jonge A, Teunissen TA, Lagro-Janssen AL. "Supine position compared to other positions during the second stage of labor: a meta-analytic review." *Journal of Psychosomatic Obstetrics and Gynecology*. 25.1 (2004:35-45. PMC. Web. 2 July 2015.

Gupta JK, Hofmeyr GJ, Smyth RMD. "Position in the second stage of labour for women without epidural anaesthesia" *Cochrane Database of Systemic Reviews*. Issue 1 (2004) Art. No. CD002006. DOI: 10.1002/14651858.CD002006.pub2.

    ** Creates narrowest pelvic opening

Michel SC, Rake A, Treiber K, Seifert B, Chaoui R, Huch R, Marincek B, Kubik-Huch RA. "MR obstetric pelvimetry: effect of birthing position on pelvic bony dimensions." *American Journal of Roentgenology* 179.4 (2002):1063-1067. PubMC. Web. 2 July 2015.

Reitter A, Daviss BA, Bisits A, Schollenberger A, Vogl T, Herrmann E, Louwen F, Zangos S. "Does pregnancy and/or shifting positions create more room in a woman's pelvis?" *American Journal of Obstetrics and Gynecology* 211.6 (2014):662. PMC. Web. 2 July 2015.

    ** Reduces blood flow to the baby

Simkin P, and O'Hara M. "Nonpharmacologic relief of pain during labor: Systematic reviews of five methods." *American Journal of Obstetrics and Gynecology* 186.5S (2002):S131–S159. Motherfriendly.org Web. 2 July 2015.

Chapter 11: Push Instinctively

1. The opposite (directed pushing) is associated with the baby receiving less oxygen as well as with an increased risk of pelvic floor dysfunction.

Roberts J, Hanson L. "Best practices in second stage labor care: maternal bearing down and positioning." *Journal of Midwifery and Women's Health* 52.3 (2007):238-245. PMC. Web. 3 July 2015.

Schaffer JI, Bloom SL, Casey BM, McIntire DD, Nihira MA, Leveno KJ. "A randomized trial of the effects of coached vs uncoached maternal pushing during the second stage of labor on postpartum pelvic floor structure and function." *American Journal of Obstetrics and Gynecology* 192.5 (2005):1692-1696. PMC. Web. 3 July 2015.

Albers LL, Sedler KD, Bedrick EJ, Teaf D, Peralta P. "Factors related to genital tract trauma in normal spontaneous vaginal births." *Birth* 33.2 (2006):94-100. PMC. Web. 3 July 2015.

2. ** Have your caregiver apply perineal support, perhaps applying a warm compress

Aasheim V, Nilsen AB, Lukasse M, Reinar LM. "Perineal techniques during the second stage of labour for reducing perineal trauma." *Cochrane Database of Systemic Reviews*. Issue 12 (2011) Art. No. CD006672. DOI: 10.1002/14651858.CD006672.pub2.

ABOUT THE AUTHOR

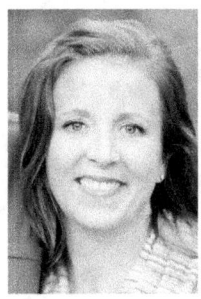

WENDY HANENBURG is the creator of the parenting website AwakeningWillow.com where her writing inspires and encourages others to create positive change in their own lives. She has written over 180 articles on topics such as healthy food, green living, mindful parenting, and, of course, natural birth.

Wendy had two natural (drug-free) births; one in a birth center, one at home, both with a midwife attending. These experiences were more powerful than she expected and led her to share the "hidden treasure" of natural birth with others.

She lives in Texas with her husband and two children. Join her at AwakeningWillow.com.